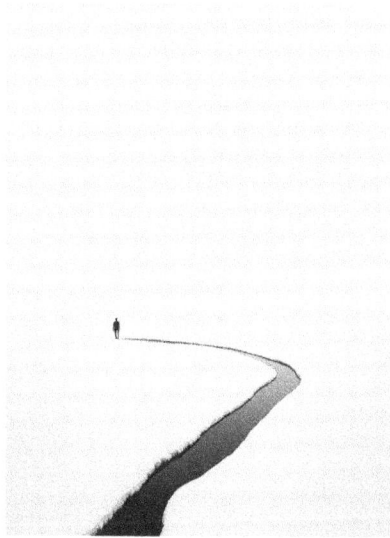

ISBN: eBook: 978-1-83990-484-4 | Paperback: 978-1-83990-482-0 | Hardcover: 978-1-83990-485-1

Introduction

About Cold Revolution

In *Cold Revolution*, we embark on a transformative journey into the fascinating intersection of cold exposure and human physiology. This ground-breaking book explores how cold immersion enhances health, mental resilience, and physical performance by tapping into the body's natural mechanisms. From vasoconstriction and shivering to the metabolic boost of burning calories to stay warm, *Cold Revolution* unpacks the science behind how the body responds to cold and how these responses can be optimized for well-being.

The book highlights a wealth of health benefits from cold exposure, including improved insulin sensitivity, reduced inflammation, and enhanced cardiovascular health. It reveals how cold therapy stimulates the production of cold shock proteins, offering potential protection against neurodegenerative diseases like Alzheimer's. Beyond the physical, cold exposure profoundly impacts mental health, reducing stress, alleviating depression, and fostering resilience by encouraging individuals to embrace and overcome discomfort.

For fitness enthusiasts, *Cold Revolution* offers insights into how cold exposure enhances endurance, accelerates recovery, and boosts athletic performance, particularly in challenging conditions. Practical guidance is provided for integrating cold therapy into daily life, whether through cold-water swimming, cold plunges, or simply adjusting home temperatures to harness its benefits.

Recognizing that individual responses to cold vary, the book examines how factors like gender, age, and body composition influence outcomes. This personalization ensures that readers can adopt safe and effective strategies tailored to their unique needs. Special attention is given to the growing practice of cold-water swimming, showcasing its mood-enhancing effects, potential metabolic benefits, and essential safety techniques.

With over 40 referenced studies, *Cold Revolution* serves as a scientifically grounded and inspiring guide for anyone curious about unlocking the body's potential. Whether you're seeking improved health, greater mental resilience, or an innovative approach to well-being, this book equips you with the knowledge to thrive in the cold and beyond.

Key Benefits from Reading this Book:

1. Boost Your Health: Learn how cold exposure improves metabolism, insulin sensitivity, and heart health.

2. Strengthen Your Mind: Discover how cold therapy reduces stress, eases depression, and builds resilience.

3. Protect Your Brain: Explore research on cold shock proteins and their role in preventing neurodegenerative diseases.

4. Optimize Fitness: Enhance endurance, speed up recovery, and perform better in cold conditions.

5. Take Action: Get practical, step-by-step methods for safely adding cold exposure to your routine.

About the Author

Andrew Bromley, an MBA graduate from the University of Birmingham, England, is a seasoned publishing professional with over 20 years of experience, including key roles at Cambridge University Press. He is also an avid triathlete, cold-water swimmer, and outdoor enthusiast.

Free Updates

Stay up to date with the latest advancements in cold therapy science. Enjoy free lifetime updates as new research emerges, keeping you informed and ahead.

Contents

Chapter One

Embracing the Cold

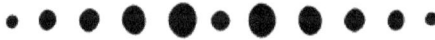

• • • ● ● • ● ● • ●

The Science and Benefits of Cold Adaptation

T he human body is an extraordinary feat of biological engineer-
ing, meticulously designed to maintain a core temperature of
approximately 37°C (98.6°F). This precise internal thermostat is essential as even slight deviations can significantly impact bodily functions.
When exposed to cold environments—from a frosty winter morning
to a briskly air-conditioned room—our bodies activate a sophisticated
suite of physiological mechanisms. These mechanisms kick in even at
the relatively mild chill of 15°C (59°F), showcasing the body's sensitive
and adaptable nature.

The strategic management of blood circulation forms one of the primary defences against the cold. Blood flow is cleverly diverted from the
extremities, such as the hands and feet, towards the core. This crucial adaptation minimizes heat loss. Consequently, blood vessels in peripheral areas
undergo vasoconstriction, reducing blood flow to these colder parts and
decreasing the surface area through which heat can escape. This redirection

often leads to a familiar sensation of numbness in these areas—a direct testament to the body's efforts to conserve heat.

As exposure to the cold extends, the body introduces additional defensive strategies to maintain its thermal equilibrium. Shivering, a widely recognized involuntary mechanism, generates heat through rapid muscular contractions. This phenomenon of shivering is not merely a reflex to cold but a complex thermogenic process. The rapid contraction and relaxation of muscles produce heat as a by-product of increased metabolic activity. Remarkably, this process can elevate the body's surface temperature in a relatively short amount of time.

The metabolic implications of shivering are profound. The calories burned during this intense muscular activity, whether derived from sugars or fats, depend on the individual's nutritional state—whether they are fasted or fed. In a fasted state, the body may break down stored fats into fatty acids, which are then oxidized to produce heat. Conversely, in a fed state, glucose from recent meals may be utilized. Thus, cold exposure not only tests our physical resilience but also presents a unique opportunity to enhance metabolic health and potentially assist in weight management.

Moreover, this adaptive response to cold exposure extends beyond mere survival; it can be harnessed for health optimization. Regular, controlled exposure to cold has been demonstrated to improve insulin sensitivity, reduce inflammation, and enhance lipid profiles by increasing levels of 'good' HDL cholesterol. These changes reflect deeper metabolic adaptations that offer long-term benefits and contribute to overall metabolic health.

Practices like cold-water immersion therapy, commonly known as "cold plunging" is an ancient restorative technique which is gaining modern-day traction for its myriad health benefits. Typically, this involves submerging most of your body, up to the shoulder girdle, in an ice bath maintained between 8-15°C (50-59°F)—akin to taking a bath in very cold water.

Immersing oneself in such an ice bath subjects the body to thermodynamic stress like that experienced in extreme cold environments. This sudden drop in temperature triggers a fight-or-flight response mediated by the autonomic (sympathetic) nervous system, signalling the body's primary focus on survival. This rapid adaptation includes a vasoconstrictive response, which increases blood pressure and shifts blood flow from the skin and extremities toward vital organs like the heart, brain, and liver to stabilize core body temperature. While this may sound daunting, when performed safely, cold-water immersion serves as a robust training regimen for the autonomic nervous system, akin to how muscles require stress to grow and strengthen.

The benefits of cold plunging extend far beyond immediate physiological responses. It has shown promise in enhancing mental resilience and alleviating stress and anxiety [1]. Regular cold plunges train the brain and body to manage acute stress more effectively. Furthermore, this practice can mitigate the inflammatory response to exercise, improve lymphatic circulation, and aid in the elimination of biological waste products from tissues and organs. These benefits can reduce delayed-onset muscle soreness, lessen feelings of fatigue, and decrease recovery times between intense physical activities [2] [3].

Understanding the Risks

As we delve into the transformative power of embracing the cold and its health benefits, it's essential to recognize that this book, like all health-related literature, offers general guidance and cannot fully address individual medical needs or evaluate specific risks related to age, pre-existing health conditions, or personal health history. Therefore, it is imperative to consult with a medical professional before undertaking any new health regimen, including cold therapy. A healthcare provider can assess its appropriateness and safety tailored to your unique health profile, ensuring that the practices you choose to engage in are beneficial and not detrimental to your well-being.

In addition to professional medical advice, paying close attention to your body's signals and responses is crucial. Everyone's physical reaction to cold exposure can vary significantly, with factors such as age, fitness level, and tolerance to cold playing significant roles. Adjust your exposure gradually to ensure comfort and safety and be mindful of any adverse reactions. If you experience any discomfort or symptoms such as excessive shivering, numbness beyond temporary tingling, or heightened stress, it's important to reassess your approach and seek medical advice.

Exercise responsibility in your cold exposure practices by adhering to recommended guidelines. Avoid excessive or prolonged exposure and ensure proper preparation and supervision where necessary. Cold exposure, when practiced responsibly, can be integrated safely into your routine to harness its benefits such as enhanced metabolic function, improved immune response, and increased mental resilience.

We invite you to join us on this journey to discover the extensive benefits that the cold can offer. By exploring and responsibly integrating cold exposure techniques in to your life, you can embark on a path toward greater resilience, vitality, and overall well-being. This journey is not just about confronting the cold but about unlocking a potent tool for health and vitality that aligns with your body's natural strengths and capabilities.

Safeguarding in Cold Environments

The ability of the human body to adapt to colder climates is not just a testament to our evolutionary resilience but also a critical mechanism for maintaining health in diverse environments. By understanding and respecting these natural responses, we can better prepare for and thrive in cold conditions, ensuring that our body's internal mechanisms are supported rather than overwhelmed.

This sophisticated understanding of the body's response to cold not only enriches our knowledge of human physiology but also underscores the importance of dressing appropriately in cold weather, engaging in proper warm-up activities before physical exertion in chilly conditions, and recognizing the signs of inadequate thermal regulation, such as prolonged numbness or ceaseless shivering, which may require medical attention. As we explore further, the ability to harness these responses healthily and effectively can open new dimensions in personal health management, from therapeutic applications like cold therapy to everyday lifestyle choices that enhance metabolic health and overall well-being.

• • • ● • ● • ● • • •

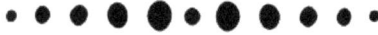

Practical Lessons from Embracing the Cold:

- **The Body Naturally Adapts to Cold:** Vasoconstriction helps retain core heat, while shivering generates energy through muscle contractions.

- **Cold-Water Therapy Offers Significant Benefits:** It boosts stress resilience, reduces inflammation, improves recovery, and enhances circulation.

- **Safe and Gradual Exposure Builds Resilience:** Responsible practices like "cold plunging" can improve both physical and mental health over time.

- **Practical Tips for Daily Cold Exposure:** Proper clothing, effective warm-up routines, and recognizing symptoms of overexposure are essential for safety.

- **Long-Term Benefits of Cold Exposure:** Regular practice strengthens immunity, boosts metabolism, and enhances overall vitality and well-being.

Chapter Two

Transformative Effects of the Cold

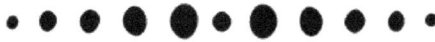

• • • ● ● • ● ● • •

Physiological Changes in a Cooler Environment

In the previous chapter, we established the remarkable capacity of the human body to maintain a core temperature of approximately 37°C (98.6°F), a prerequisite for sustaining essential physiological processes. When the body encounters cooler temperatures, even as mild as 15°C (59°F), it initiates a sophisticated array of physiological responses tailored to preserve this vital temperature range.

One of the cornerstone responses to cold exposure is the strategic redistribution of blood flow, a phenomenon known as vasoconstriction. This process involves the narrowing of blood vessels, particularly those in the peripheral regions such as the hands, feet, and skin surface. By constricting these vessels, the body minimizes heat loss and redirects warmer blood towards the core, where it is critically needed. This process can inadvertently aid in weight management, as the body consumes energy stored in fat to fuel the shivering process. This aspect of cold exposure can be particularly appealing to those looking to manage their weight effectively, making shivering a useful albeit involuntary exercise mechanism.

When you next experience numbness in your extremities or the onset of shivering, take a moment to appreciate the complexity and efficiency of your body's thermal regulation system. This system does not merely react passively to changes in environmental temperatures but actively manages your internal climate to ensure that vital functions are maintained. It acts as a sophisticated internal thermostat, prioritizing and protecting your essential organs through intricate and dynamic adjustments that are fundamental to survival.

Hypothermia Prevention

This shift in blood flow is essential for preventing hypothermia, a potentially fatal condition. It can impair neurological and muscular functions, leading to lethargy and a weakened heartbeat, significantly risking organ failure and, if unaddressed, death. The body's ability to restrict peripheral blood flow and concentrate warmth centrally is therefore a critical survival strategy in cold environments.

Shivering: A Dual-Purpose Mechanism

The body initiates shivering as a rapid, involuntary contraction of muscles, serving as an efficient mechanism to generate heat and maintain body temperature. Shivering serves a dual purpose: it helps to maintain the core temperature at a stable level and acts as a metabolic booster. Although often perceived as merely uncomfortable, shivering is an efficient process for heat production. The rapid twitching of muscles during shivering generates significant amounts of heat, akin to how a space heater warms a chilly room.

In addition to heat production, shivering has a beneficial side effect on metabolism. This intense muscular activity requires energy, thus burning calories at an accelerated rate. This increased metabolic rate may have a beneficial effect on metabolic health.

Could a Cooler Room Lower Your Risk of Type 2 Diabetes?

The assertion that adjusting your thermostat could play a role in preventing type 2 diabetes is indeed a bold and somewhat controversial one to make. However, this question serves as a thought-provoking introduction to a nuanced discussion based on emerging scientific research that we will explore throughout the book.

Scientific Foundations

Recent studies suggest a link between ambient temperature and diabetes risk. Lowering the thermostat during colder months may potentially reduce the risk of developing type 2 diabetes, as suggested by preliminary research [1]. This connection is believed to stem from the body's metabolic response to cooler temperatures, which can activate processes beneficial for glucose regulation and overall metabolic health.

In a controlled study, participants were exposed to a cooler environment of 15°C (59°F) for six hours each day over a span of ten days. This exposure led to significant improvements in how their bodies processed glucose. Specifically, participants showed up to a 40% improvement in their ability to regulate blood glucose levels after this period of cold exposure. The underlying mechanism for this improvement is linked to an increase in the activity of Glucose Transporter Type 4 (GLUT4), a protein essential for transporting glucose from the bloodstream into the muscles, where it can be used for energy rather than being stored as fat.

Additionally, the process of adapting to colder temperatures was found to not only enhance glucose metabolism but also reduce overall cholesterol and blood pressure levels. These benefits underscore the body's adaptive responses to cold, which appear to extend beyond simple thermal regulation to encompass broader metabolic improvements.

The mechanisms by which mild cold exposure might mitigate diabetes risk include increased energy expenditure and enhanced utilization of glucose and fatty acids. These effects improve insulin sensitivity and fasting glucose levels in healthy individuals, indicating a preventive potential against metabolic diseases driven by energy mismanagement, such as obesity and type 2 diabetes. As a disease, type 2 diabetes is increasingly prevalent worldwide, influenced by a complex interplay of factors including genetics, dietary habits, meal frequency, and sedentary lifestyles. In this context, every potential preventive measure deserves consideration, particularly those that might integrate seamlessly into our daily lives.

Practical Applications and Lifestyle Integration

For those considering this approach, it is essential to integrate gradual temperature adjustments thoughtfully within the broader context of a healthy lifestyle. Begin by slightly lowering your thermostat and carefully observing how your body responds. This cautious approach not only aids in acclimatization but also maximizes the health benefits without introducing undue stress or discomfort.

Fat Metabolism and Brown Adipose Tissue

The human body hosts a variety of fat cells, each type performing unique and critical roles in our metabolic health. One of the key distinctions in our understanding of fat involves the difference between white adipose tissue (often simply referred to as body fat) and brown adipose tissue (BAT), also known as brown fat. Recent advancements in medical research have shed light on how exposure to cooler environments can significantly influence the amount and activity of brown fat, which is increasingly recognized for its beneficial roles in energy metabolism and potential in weight management strategies.

Brown fat is uniquely equipped with a high number of mitochondria, the "powerhouses" of cells, which contain iron—giving the tissue its characteristic brown colour. This type of fat is metabolically active and plays a crucial role in thermogenesis, the process of heat production in organisms. From birth, infants have significant amounts of brown fat located primarily behind their shoulder blades. This is vital for infants, who are less capable of shivering—a natural response to cold in older children and adults that also generates heat. The strategic placement of brown fat, deep in the body around the shoulder blades, spine, and kidneys, not only facilitates heat production but also protects and maintains the temperature of vital organs.

Contrary to previous beliefs that brown fat was only significant in infants, recent studies have shown that adults also retain active brown fat. More intriguingly, the levels and activity of brown fat can be increased through exposure to cooler environments—a process sometimes referred to as "cold therapy." This discovery marks a significant shift in how we might approach conditions like obesity and metabolic syndrome, as increased brown fat activity correlates with enhanced energy expenditure and potentially improved weight management.

Further research has illuminated that brown fat in adults is not just residual but actively participates in energy metabolism [2]. When adults are exposed to cold temperatures, their brown fat activates, burning calories to generate heat. This process significantly impacts overall energy balance and can influence body weight and metabolic health. Studies have documented that even mild stimulation of brown fat activity through exposure to cooler temperatures can improve insulin sensitivity and glucose metabolism, which are crucial for overall metabolic health.

Potential for Combating Metabolic Disorders

The capacity of brown fat to convert energy into heat, a process known as non-shivering thermogenesis, suggests a promising avenue for the treatment and prevention of obesity and related metabolic disorders. Increasing the activity of brown fat could lead to substantial improvements in the body's ability to process glucose and fats, potentially reducing the risk of developing type 2 diabetes and other metabolic conditions.

While the benefits of activating brown fat through cold exposure are compelling, more research is necessary to fully understand the mechanisms and optimize methods for safely harnessing this potential. The impact of brown fat on overall metabolic health is a dynamic area of study that promises to offer new insights into how we might better manage and prevent common metabolic health issues in the future.

Differences Between the Sexes in Cold Perception

Have you ever found yourself in a "heated" debate over the seemingly simple question of whether it's cold enough to turn on the heating at home or adjust the air conditioning in the office? It's a common scenario, with discussions often becoming unexpectedly spirited as each party believes the other is being unreasonable. The crux of these disagreements might stem from a fundamental difference in how men and women perceive and react to cold temperatures

Gender Differences in Thermal Perception

Scientific studies have documented that men and women can experience temperature differently. These differences are attributed to variations in body composition, such as muscle mass and fat distribution, which affect how heat is produced and retained in the body [3]. Typically, men possess greater muscle mass, which acts as an insulator and generates more body heat, thus providing better natural insulation. In contrast, women might start to feel cold and may even begin to shiver at temperatures approximately 4°C (39°F) higher than those at which men would typically feel cold. This disparity can significantly impact comfort levels in shared environments like homes and offices, making a one-size-fits-all temperature setting challenging to achieve.

Further insights into gender-specific responses to cold come from studies on brown adipose tissue. Women generally have higher quantities of brown fat compared to men and are more adept at activating it in response to cold [4]. This type of fat is metabolically active, capable of burning calories to generate heat. The enhanced ability to activate brown fat might also contribute to metabolic advantages in women, such as a potentially lower risk for developing type 2 diabetes, as brown fat helps to improve insulin sensitivity and glucose metabolism.

Implications for Everyday Life

Understanding these physiological differences is more than an academic exercise; it has practical implications for daily life. For instance, recognizing that women might require warmer temperatures to feel comfortable can help in setting thermostats in shared spaces to accommodate everyone's comfort.

Here are some strategies to manage differing temperature needs effectively:

Gradual Temperature Reduction

- To accommodate varying thermal preferences, start by slightly lowering the heating settings and observe how each person reacts. Gradual changes can help the body adjust without causing discomfort.

Embrace Mild Cold

- Experiencing mild cold can be beneficial. It does not require extreme temperature drops but rather small adjustments that can activate the body's adaptive mechanisms, leading to improved health outcomes.

Account for Others

- Always consider the comfort and health implications for all individuals in a shared space, especially those who may be more vulnerable to cold, such as the elderly or those with chronic health issues.

Consult a Healthcare Professional

- Before implementing any significant changes to how you manage temperature at home or in the workplace, especially for those with pre-existing health conditions, consulting with a healthcare provider is advisable.

By understanding how different bodies react to cold, we can foster environments that are not only physically comfortable but also supportive of metabolic health and well-being. The subsequent sections of this book will delve into detailed methods of cold exposure and explore their impacts on health and vitality. As we proceed, we invite you to join us on a journey toward increased resilience and enhanced well-being through the transformative effects of cold exposure.

• • • ● ● • ● ● • • •

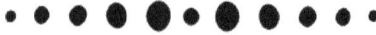

Practical Lessons from Transformative Effects of the Cold:

- **Adaptive Physiological Mechanisms**: The body's response to cold includes vasoconstriction, shivering, and hormonal adjustments, which help maintain core temperature and enhance survival.

- **Health Advantages**: Cold exposure can improve metabolic health, activate brown fat, and boost cardiovascular function.

- **Implementation Strategies**: Safe practices include gradual adaptation, consultation with healthcare professionals, and integration with a holistic health approach.

- **Scientific Evidence**: Initial studies suggest the benefits of mild cold exposure in improving glucose metabolism and reducing the risk of type 2 diabetes but more research is needed in this area to back up these early findings .

- **Personalized Approaches**: Consider gender-specific physiological responses to tailor cold exposure practices to individual needs.

Chapter Three

Winter Wellness

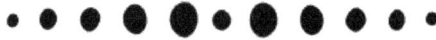

• • ● ● ● • ● ● • •

Advantages of Winter Workouts

T his section explores the link between the colder months and a de-
cline in physical activity, illustrating how reversing this trend can
significantly elevate your fitness regimen. We highlight the unique benefits
of winter exercise, supported by contemporary research which posits that
cooler conditions may enable more intense and vigorous training sessions.
We delve into the physiological mechanisms that allow your body to perform optimally in cold weather and discuss the ideal temperature ranges
that maximize workout benefits. Practical advice is also provided to help
you capitalize on the brisk outdoor temperatures to enhance your fitness
outcomes.

Recent meta-analyses that review a broad spectrum of studies on temperature and athletic performance robustly support the idea that colder conditions can improve running efficiency [1]. It has been found that the optimal temperature for individuals who typically run a mile in 9 minutes or longer is between 10°C (50°F) and 11°C (51.8°F). For more experienced runners, those capable of completing a mile in less than 9 minutes, even colder temperatures—ranging from 4°C (39.2°F) to 8°C (46.4°F)—may be preferable. This specific range is often referred to as the "Goldilocks Zone" for physically fit adults but why does cooler weather provide such benefits?

The advantages of exercising during cooler months are deeply rooted in the fundamentals of human physiology: cooler temperatures help prevent the body from overheating. This regulation aids in conserving energy that would otherwise be expended on thermoregulation—actively cooling down. This conservation allows athletes to sustain higher levels of exertion for longer periods without succumbing to early fatigue. Additionally, exercising in cooler conditions can increase the efficiency of oxygen uptake, further enhancing endurance and performance.

However, cold-weather exercise also presents unique challenges. One must be vigilant about the potential dangers such as frostbite and slippery conditions due to ice, which are more prevalent as temperatures drop. These hazards require increased caution and preparedness to ensure safety during workouts.

Furthermore, it is crucial to consult with a healthcare provider before engaging in cold-weather exercise, especially for those with pre-existing medical conditions or concerns about the impact of cold on their health. This precautionary step ensures that individuals can safely maximize the benefits of their winter exercise regime.

By fully understanding these dynamics and preparing adequately, the winter months can be transformed into a productive period for enhancing physical fitness. This can lead to improved overall health and athletic performance. In the subsequent sections, we will delve deeper into selecting the appropriate gear, developing effective warm-up routines, and implementing recovery strategies specifically tailored for cold-weather workouts. These guidelines will equip you to pursue your fitness goals robustly, even as temperatures plummet, ensuring that you remain well-prepared to tackle any challenges posed by the colder climate.

The Science Behind Exercising in the Cold

The cooler your body temperature, the less blood needs to circulate to your skin to dissipate heat, a natural response when overheating occurs. Consequently, during intense physical activities like running and cycling, maintaining a cooler body temperature can result in a lower heart rate. This reduced cardiac demand enables you to sustain higher workout intensities with less strain on your heart. However, it's important to recognize that not all forms of exercise benefit equally from cooler temperatures. For example, sprinting, which relies on short, intense bursts of energy, may experience reduced performance in colder conditions as muscles do not warm up as efficiently [2] . Furthermore, in relation to muscle growth, for example within the context of power, and body building, there is a debate within the scientific community about the precise impact of cold on muscle hypertrophy. Some studies suggest that training in cold conditions can lead to less effective muscular contractions and possibly a higher risk of injury due to reduced elasticity in muscles and connective tissue. Other research, however, indicates that with proper warm-up and adaptation, the effects can be mitigated.

Additionally, exercising in cold weather can increase the production of cytokines, signalling molecules released by muscles and fat tissue. These cytokines provide various health benefits. A notable example is Irisin, a cytokine that is activated both by physical exertion and exposure to cold temperatures. A small study has indicated that cold-weather workouts can boost the production of Irisin by nearly 20% [3]. This is particularly significant because Irisin plays a crucial role in regulating blood glucose levels and maintaining cardiovascular health . While more research is needed to fully understand these effects, initial findings suggest that winter workouts could offer additional cardiovascular benefits and assist in glucose regulation, which is particularly advantageous for individuals with type 2 diabetes or elevated blood glucose levels.

The psychological benefits of cold-weather training also merit attention. The brisk feel of cooler air and the captivating beauty of winter landscapes can greatly enhance mood and mental well-being. This aesthetic appeal, combined with the physical advantages, often leads to more consistent engagement with exercise routines during the winter months. Research indicates that the natural light and visual stimuli associated with outdoor winter activities can help alleviate symptoms of seasonal affective disorder (SAD), offering both psychological and physiological benefits. Thus, embracing outdoor activities in colder weather not only invigorates your fitness regimen but also boosts your overall health and wellness, presenting a robust option for those aiming to optimize their fitness outcomes throughout the year.

The Physiological Effects of the Cold on Your Body

Stepping outside on a crisp winter's day, the cold is palpable, biting at your face and hands. Your body reacts instinctively to this sharp cold stimulus, launching a series of physiological changes aimed at preserving core warmth. It achieves this by diverting blood flow away from the extremities, especially those exposed areas like fingers and toes, and redirecting it towards the core. This safeguarding measure is vital as it helps maintain the temperature of your vital organs, preventing them from cooling down excessively. During this process, the peripheral blood vessels constrict, a phenomenon known as vasoconstriction, which intensifies the blood flow to the core while reducing it at the surface of the skin. This adjustment can lead to a numbing and sometimes semi-painful sensation in your fingertips and other extremities, signalling that your body's thermal regulatory system is actively working to keep your internal temperature steady at an optimal range.

While the body's response to cold is a marvel of human physiology, prolonged exposure to extreme cold is dangerous. Extended periods in such conditions can lead to a significant drop in body temperature, at which point the heart, nervous system, and other vital organs begin to function abnormally. However, moderate exposure to cold while being active can be beneficial. Movement generates body heat, which helps mitigate the initial discomfort of the cold. Blood gradually returns to the extremities, warming them and providing relief from the initial cold-induced numbness.

Exploring further the benefits of exercising in cooler conditions, let us compare this to working out in warmer weather. On a pleasantly warm day, say between 25 to 30°C (77° to 86°F), your cardiovascular system is under considerable stress. Your heart beats vigorously to pump blood not only to the muscles, which demand more oxygen during exercise, but also to the skin to help dissipate the additional heat generated by physical activity. This dual demand increases cardiovascular strain, compounded by significant sweating—potentially up to 2 litres per hour—which can quickly lead to dehydration. If your body cannot efficiently manage the heat through sufficient blood flow to the skin or adequate sweating, physical performance is compromised, necessitating a slowdown or complete cessation of activity.

In contrast, cooler weather, particularly in the range of 10 to 11°C (50° to 52°F), presents a more favourable condition for physical exertion. The wider gap between your internal body temperature and the external temperature allows for more efficient heat loss, which means less blood needs to be diverted to the skin and more remains available for your muscles and cardiovascular system. This allows for prolonged activity at a higher intensity with increased fitness benefits. Nonetheless, caution is advised in temperatures below 10°C (50°F), especially for those not accustomed to cold weather exercise. At these lower temperatures, muscle and nerve efficiency at the extremities can be compromised, which may impede your ability to perform physical tasks effectively. Moreover, individuals with conditions such as asthma may find cold and dry air exacerbates their symptoms, necessitating additional precautions during cold weather activities.

In general, the research consistently demonstrates that exercise in cooler environments can help with performance for more aerobic exercises, especially running. For those who live in warmer climates or want the benefits in the summer months than cold-water immersion can significantly improve performance [4][5]. Cold plunging before a workout may also produce an acute increase in metabolic rate and reduce the perception of pain and exertion during exercise, but it's unclear if this results in substantial long-term benefits.

What to Wear

When preparing to exercise in cold weather, dressing appropriately is crucial for comfort and safety. The art of layering cannot be overstated—it allows for adjustable insulation and breathability, adapting as your body temperature fluctuates with activity levels. Start with a moisture-wicking base layer to keep sweat away from your skin, preventing a chill. Add a thermal middle layer for insulation, which can be adjusted based on how cold it is. Your outer layer should be wind and water-resistant, protecting you from the elements.

For individuals with specific medical conditions like Raynaud's, protective, and insulated gloves and socks are vital. These accessories should be thick enough to retain heat but not so bulky as to restrict movement. Similarly, those with heart conditions or other serious health concerns should always consult their doctor before beginning an exercise routine, especially in cold weather. Start slowly and increase the intensity gradually, always mindful of your body's responses to the new stresses.

· • ● ● ● • ● ● • • ·

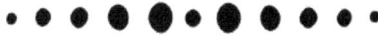

Practical Lessons from Winter Wellness:

- **Cardiovascular Health Benefits:** Exercising in cold weather can be beneficial for your heart and blood vessels. The lower temperatures help reduce the strain on your heart that would normally be used for cooling down your body, allowing it to work more efficiently.

- **Easier on Your Cardiovascular System:** For many, colder weather allows for longer, more comfortable workouts as the heart does not need to work as hard to cool the body down. This can also mean the potential to push harder during workouts, increasing intensity without overheating.

- **Enjoy the Outdoors:** Cold weather workouts provide a unique opportunity to enjoy the outdoors during all seasons. Whether it's the serene silence after a snowfall or the crisp air of a winter morning, exercising outside can refresh your mind as well as your body.

- **Boost to Your Immune System:** Regular exercise is a proven immune system booster, and doing so in the cold may amplify this effect. The cold environment itself has been shown to stimulate the immune response, potentially increasing your body's ability toward off illnesses.

- **Mental Health Advantages:** Exercising outdoors during the colder months can also combat seasonal affective disorder (SAD), a type of depression that typically occurs during the winter. Exposure to natural light, even in reduced amounts, can help mitigate some of the symptoms associated with this condition.

- **Adaptability and Resilience:** Acclimating to the cold for regular workouts can help develop a stronger tolerance to adverse conditions, enhancing your physical resilience. This adaptability can translate to improved performance and endurance, beneficial for both everyday activities and competitive sports.

By embracing these practices, you can transform the cold months into a period of significant health and fitness gains. Dressing appropriately, understanding the specific needs of your health condition, and gradually adapting to the colder temperatures can help you maintain a safe and effective workout regime throughout the year.

Chapter Four

Cold Water Swimming

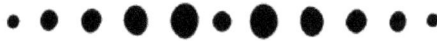

• • • ● • ● ● • • •

The Healing Powers of Cold-Water Swimming

In recent years, the invigorating practice of winter swimming, also known as cold-water swimming, has surged in popularity globally. As a form of physical and mental challenge, enthusiasts brave the chilling waters of lakes, rivers, seas, and outdoor pools, even during the harshest winter months. This growing trend is not just about enduring the cold; it's increasingly seen as a therapeutic ritual, with a compelling array of potential health benefits that are capturing the attention of both the public and scientific communities.

Emerging research suggests that immersing oneself in cold water can do more than just invigorate the spirit; it may also offer significant physiological benefits. Key among these are enhancements in mood and energy levels. The shock of cold water triggers a flood of mood-lifting neurotransmitters, making swimmers feel more vibrant and alert. Additionally, there's evidence to suggest that cold water immersion can reduce inflammation, potentially offering relief from muscle soreness and joint pain, which is a boon for athletes and those with chronic pain conditions.

Moreover, recent studies indicate potential metabolic benefits, including improved blood sugar regulation. This is particularly significant given the rising rates of metabolic syndromes globally. The mechanisms behind these effects are still under investigation, but they may relate to the body's heightened metabolic rate as it works to generate warmth in response to cold exposure.

Perhaps most intriguing is the preliminary research pointing to neuroprotective effects. Scientists are exploring how cold-water swimming could release a specific protein known to protect against neurodegeneration. This has profound implications for diseases like Alzheimer's and other forms of dementia. If substantiated, such findings could revolutionize approaches to neurodegenerative disease prevention and therapy.

In this chapter, we will delve deeper into the scientific literature surrounding cold-water swimming. We'll explore the known physiological responses to cold exposure, discuss the latest research findings, and consider the anecdotal evidence provided by a global community of cold-water swimmers. Each section will include a discussion of the strengths and limitations of current studies, and where the scientific community calls for further inquiry to solidify these promising findings.

As we unpack the science and stories behind this chilling yet exhilarating practice, we aim to provide a balanced view, acknowledging where the evidence is strong and where questions remain. By the end of this chapter, you should have a clearer understanding of why plunging into icy waters might be more than just a test of endurance—it could be a key to better health and longevity.

Cold Water Swimming and Mental Health Relief

The relationship between cold-water swimming and mental health, particularly its potential effects on depression, has garnered attention both anecdotally and in scientific circles. Numerous personal accounts suggest that cold-water immersion can significantly alleviate symptoms associated with depression, including those linked to chronic pain. Additionally, specific demographic groups, such as women undergoing menopause, have reported a notable decrease in their symptoms, prompting questions about the underlying mechanisms: Is this merely a placebo effect, or does cold-water swimming offer genuine therapeutic benefits?

One compelling case study from the UK featured a 24-year-old woman who had been struggling with major depressive disorder and anxiety, necessitating continuous medical treatment for over seven years. According to a report [1], as part of her treatment, she initiated a regimen of supervised cold-water swimming once a week. Remarkably, within a month, she was able to taper off her medication, and after four months, she discontinued her pharmacological treatment altogether [2]. While this case is inspiring, it also prompts caution; individual results can vary significantly, and multiple factors could contribute to such positive outcomes, necessitating a careful evaluation of causality.

Further reinforcing these individual narratives, a larger-scale study surveyed over 700 outdoor swimmers [3]. The findings echoed the anecdotal evidence, showing marked improvements in mood and over-all mental well-being among the participants. This study suggests that physical activity, particularly in the form of cold-water swimming, might play a role in enhancing mental health and reducing symptoms of various psychological disorders.

However, it is crucial to note that while these studies provide valu-able insights, they do not establish a definitive relationship between cold-water swimming and improvements in mental health. The cur-rent research primarily offers correlations that invite deeper investiga-tion into the physiological and psychological mechanisms at play.

We will explore the potential biochemical and neuroendocrine re-sponses triggered by cold-water immersion that could explain its an-tidepressant effects and delve into theories regarding how cold stress might increase the production of endorphins, enhance neurotransmit-ter function, or reset stress response systems in the brain. Additionally, we will examine the role of the 'cold shock' proteins and their possible impact on brain health.

By reviewing the potential of cold-water swimming as a non-pharma-ceutical intervention for depression, weaving together scientific research, case studies, and survey data to offer a well-rounded perspective. While highlighting the promising therapeutic benefits, it also acknowledges the current research limitations and underscores the need for robust clinical trials to further validate its efficacy. Through this exploration, readers will gain a nuanced understanding of cold-water swimming—not merely as a physical feat, but as a transformative approach that could open new pathways for mental health treatment and holistic well-being.

The Neuroprotective Benefits of Cold-Water Swimming

In the emerging field of study surrounding the physiological and psychological benefits of cold-water swimming, there remains no absolute consensus. However, a growing body of research suggests plausible mechanistic processes that may underpin the myriads of benefits reported. The principal theory posits significant alterations in blood flow—most notably within cerebral regions associated with mood regulation. This hypothesis is bolstered by a landmark study [4], which recorded enhancements in blood sugar control and insulin sensitivity over a six-month period. It's important to note that these benefits were specifically observed in women with lower body fat percentages.

Further research highlights the potential health benefits linked to regular cold-water immersion. For instance, habitual outdoor swimmers exhibited a 40% reduced likelihood of contracting respiratory tract infections (RTIs), encompassing a range of ailments from the common cold to acute otitis media [5]. Such infections can affect both the upper respiratory tract—including the nose, nasal cavity, and pharynx—and the lower respiratory tract, which includes the larynx, trachea, bronchi, and lungs.

The underlying mechanisms appear to stem largely from the body's initial shock response upon entering cold water. This response triggers a cascade of physiological changes: an involuntary gasp followed by rapid breathing, spikes in heart rate and blood pressure, and substantial redistributions of blood flow from the skin to the body's core. These changes are primarily driven by efforts to maintain core body temperature. Concurrently, there is a surge in stress-related hormones such as adrenaline, noradrenaline, and cortisol. These chemicals heighten alertness and readiness, propelling the body into a fight-or-flight state within milliseconds.

As the cold shock response abates and breathing normalizes, which can take several minutes, the individual is prepared to swim. The release of stress hormones during this phase is thought to positively influence mood and potentially alleviate symptoms of depression. This effect is attributed to 'cross adaptation,' where the body's adjustment to the cold-water stressor may enhance its overall resilience to other life stresses.

The challenge of cold-water immersion is daunting, yet overcoming this fear and adapting to the cold confers psychological benefits, priming individuals for other life challenges. Additionally, the communal aspect of group swimming offers not only safety but also enriches social interactions, further contributing to the physiological advantages of this activity.

Over time, as one becomes acclimatized to cold-water conditions, the initial intense responses—like the shock and rapid breathing—tend to diminish significantly, evidenced by up to a 50% reduction in breathing rate and a lower heart rate. Notably, even after periods of cessation, the adaptation benefits appear to persist, suggesting a lasting impact of cold-water swimming on the body's baseline state [6].

While more research is required to fully elucidate the adaptation benefits and potential enhancements to protein expression associated with cold-water swimming, the existing scientific literature indicates a substantial and multifaceted impact on health.

Cold Shock Proteins in Neurodegenerative Therapy

RMB3, which stands for RNA-binding motif protein 3, is a type of cold shock protein that is particularly notable for its response to low temperature stress in cells. It belongs to a broader class of proteins known as RNA-binding proteins, which play critical roles in various cellular processes by interacting with RNA to influence its function.

In the context of human health and disease, the study of RMB3 is relatively new but promising, particularly in the field of neurodegenerative diseases. Research has suggested that cold shock proteins like RMB3 might have neuroprotective properties. For instance, in experimental models, increased levels of such proteins have been associated with protection against neurological damage and improved outcomes in conditions like Alzheimer's disease. The hypothesis is that these proteins could help protect brain cells from the types of stress and damage typically seen in neurodegeneration. Initial studies have revealed that exposure to cold environments can activate RMB3, which subsequently makes its way to the brain via the bloodstream. This process has been shown to have beneficial effects on brain health, particularly by potentially mitigating the impacts of neurodegenerative disorders [7], [8].

Extensive research involving animal models has consistently demonstrated that by lowering body temperature, not only activates RMB3 but also increases its production. This response suggests a natural protective mechanism that could be leveraged to develop new treatments for diseases like Alzheimer's. For example, one influential study found that administering RMB3 to mice with Alzheimer's-like symptoms resulted in notable improvements, including restored memory functions. These results highlight RMB3's potential as a powerful neuroprotective agent [9].

Despite these exciting advancements, the translation of these findings to human health remains complex. Human trials have shown varying levels of RMB3 in participants engaged in cold-water swimming [10]. Some individuals show significant increases in RMB3 levels, which correlate with the neuroprotective effects observed in animal studies. However, these increases are not universal, indicating that individual genetic and physiological differences may influence the response to cold exposure.

The variability in human responses underscores the need for a deeper understanding of the mechanisms through which RMB3 operates. It is crucial to investigate how RMB3 interacts with other biological pathways and factors that influence brain health. Such research could pave the way for personalized therapeutic approaches that consider individual differences in genetic makeup and lifestyle.

Further, ethical considerations must be carefully managed, especially when moving from animal models to human trials. The potential side effects of artificially inducing cold stress or administering RMB3 directly are not yet fully understood, and rigorous clinical trials are necessary to ensure safety and efficacy.

Future research should focus on expanding the scope of clinical trials to include diverse populations to better understand the broader applicability of RMB3-based treatments. Additionally, studies should explore optimal conditions under which cold exposure can safely and effectively increase RMB3 levels in humans.

As we continue to unravel the potential of RMB3, it is also worth exploring synergistic effects with other treatments and lifestyle interventions. Could combining cold exposure with specific dietary supplements, exercise routines, or pharmacological treatments amplify the benefits of RMB3? Exploring these possibilities could lead to comprehensive treatment plans that address the multifaceted nature of neurodegenerative diseases.

While the road to clinical application is long and fraught with challenges, the promising early research into RMB3 and cold exposure offers hope for developing innovative strategies to combat some of the most debilitating health conditions. The ongoing investigation into this cold-induced protein not only advances our understanding of biological stress responses but also opens new frontiers in the treatment of neurodegenerative diseases.

Guidelines for Cold Water Swimming

Cold water swimming can be a rejuvenating and invigorating experience, offering numerous health benefits. However, it also presents unique challenges and risks, particularly for those new to the practice. If you are considering taking up cold water swimming, it's important to approach this activity with caution and proper preparation.

For beginners, the best time to start cold water swimming is not during the winter but in the warmer months. Spring or early summer offers a gentler introduction to the cooler temperatures you'll eventually face. This gradual introduction helps your body adapt to the cold more effectively, reducing the shock and stress associated with colder waters.

There is no one-size-fits-all answer to what constitutes "cold" water. Water temperature that feels chilly to one person might feel tolerable to another. Cold water swimming typically involves temperatures that can induce a cold shock response—this is the involuntary intake of breath and increased heart rate that happens when your body reacts to cold. Everyone's threshold for this response is different, which makes personal comfort and physical response important factors to consider.

Preparing Your Body – Cold Showers and Acclimatization

Before attempting to swim in cold water, it's advisable to prepare your body using cold showers. This method helps you gradually get used to the sensation of cold and can mitigate the intensity of the cold shock response when you do enter a natural body of water.

If you have any underlying health conditions, particularly cardiovascular issues, it's essential to consult with a healthcare provider before starting cold water swimming. The stress of cold water can exacerbate certain health conditions. Additionally, it's important to be aware of the risks of hypothermia, discussed previously and occurs when your body loses heat faster than it can produce it, causing a dangerous drop in body temperature.

Cold water can also affect your nerves, potentially making them stiffer and less responsive. This can impair coordination, affect your swimming stroke, and increase the risk of drowning if not managed properly. Therefore, always ensure that you are thoroughly warmed up and have recovered from the initial cold shock response before beginning to swim.

Safety in Numbers

Joining a local swimming group is highly recommended for beginners. Not only does this provide a safer environment by ensuring there are people to help in case of emergencies, but it also enhances the overall enjoyment of the activity. Swimming with others can provide motivation and make the challenging moments more manageable.

Approaching cold water swimming with careful preparation and respect for the body's responses to cold can make this activity both safe and enjoyable. Remember, gradual adaptation is key to a successful and healthful cold water swimming experience.

Cold-water swimming has captured the attention of health enthusiasts and researchers alike due to its wide range of potential health benefits. By braving chilly waters, swimmers may experience physical, psychological, and possibly neuroprotective benefits.

• • • ● • ● • ● • • •

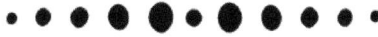

Practical Lessons from Cold Water Swimming:

- **Mood Enhancement:** One of the most immediate and noticeable benefits of cold-water swimming is the boost in mood it can provide. The shock of cold water stimulates the production of endorphins, the body's natural painkillers that also act as mood elevators. This hormonal response can lead to feelings of euphoria and general well-being, often referred to as the "swimmer's high." Regular participants report significant improvements in their mental health, including reductions in stress and anxiety.

- **Metabolic Improvement:** Cold water imposes a thermal stress on the body, which must expend more energy to maintain its core temperature. This process can boost metabolism, as the body burns more calories to generate heat. Over time, this can lead to improved metabolic efficiency, which is beneficial for overall energy levels and weight management. Additionally, some studies suggest that repeated cold exposure might promote the conversion of white fat into brown fat, the latter of which is more metabolically active and efficient at burning calories.

- **Enhanced Immune Response:** Regular cold-water swimming has been associated with an enhanced immune response. The physiological stress caused by cold exposure stimulates the immune system, potentially increasing the body's ability to fight off infections, including respiratory infections. Swimmers often report fewer colds and flu-like symptoms compared to non-swimmers, which could be attributed to this improved immune function.

- **Potential Neurological Protection:** Although still in the early stages of research, there is promising evidence to suggest that cold-water swimming may contribute to neurological health. The activity has been linked to the production of cold shock proteins such as RMB3, which have shown potential in protecting against neurodegeneration. These proteins could play a role in preventing or slowing the progression of conditions like Alzheimer's and Parkinson's disease. However, more extensive, and in-depth studies are required to fully understand this connection and its implications for long-term brain health.

Extending the Benefits Through Lifestyle Integration

Integrating cold-water swimming into a regular lifestyle regimen can enhance its benefits. To maximize these positive effects, it is recommended to combine swimming with other healthy habits, such as a balanced diet, regular exercise, and sufficient sleep. Moreover, mindfulness and relaxation techniques can complement the stress-reducing aspects of cold-water immersion, leading to a more rounded approach to mental and physical health.

Chapter Five

Getting Started – Preparing for the Cold Water

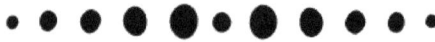

• • • • ● ● ● • • •

Essential Tips and Techniques to Brave the Chill

I n the enthralling world of cold-water swimming, the journey from the nerve-wracking first plunge to mastering this chilling sport unfolds through a series of transformative experiences. That initial dive into icy waters can indeed be daunting. As fear grips every fibre of your being, the frigid embrace feels almost overwhelming. Yet, fuelled by a mix of excitement and adrenaline, you push through, propelled by the thrill of stepping into the unknown and the raw challenge it presents.

Then comes the dreaded second swim—the novelty has now faded, and the chill cuts through you with an even sharper edge. With the element of surprise gone, you're fully aware of what awaits. This heightened awareness only intensifies your sensation of the cold. It's more than a physical test; it's a profound mental battle, challenging your resilience and determination.

By the third dip, however, a subtle yet significant transformation begins. You start to embrace the cold, surrendering to its icy grip. The initial discomfort gradually gives way to a strange sense of exhilaration. It's during these moments that you begin to understand the allure of cold-water swimming—the raw purity of the environment, the clarity it brings to your mind, and the invigorating shock to the body that somehow heightens your senses and invigorates your spirit.

Acclimatization to the cold is a gradual process. It takes time—often up to six dips, according to seasoned swimmers. Each session builds your endurance, enhances your tolerance, and deepens your connection to this extreme form of immersion. Thus, for those embarking on this icy adventure for the first time, patience and perseverance are essential. Commit to at least six swims before making any judgments on whether the brisk world of cold-water swimming is truly for you. Through persistence, what once seemed unbearably cold may soon become a refreshing and vital part of your routine, offering a unique escape and an exhilarating challenge.

At its essence, cold-water swimming is deceptively simple. It's swimming, akin to what you might do in any sun-warmed pool or balmy sea. The basic requirement is straightforward: know how to swim. Yet, beneath this façade of simplicity, a complex world of preparation and precaution unfolds—a testament to the serious nature of engaging with nature's colder elements.

Before you plunge into the realm of cold-water swimming, consider three pivotal elements that underpin a safe and enjoyable experience:

- Location and Timing: Selecting the right venue is paramount. Choose a location that not only captivates your spirit but also suits your swimming skills and goals. This could be a serene lake, a sheltered bay, or a controlled cold-water swimming facility. Consider the accessibility, safety features, and natural conditions of the spot. Aligning your swims with the right time of day can also enhance your experience, taking advantage of natural light and typically calmer waters.

- Companionship and Safety: The value of a swimming partner cannot be overstressed. Whether it's a friend or a community of cold-water enthusiasts, companions not only provide moral support but are crucial for safety. Swimming alone in cold waters increases risk significantly. A buddy system ensures that help is at hand in case of any unforeseen difficulties, and it makes the challenge more enjoyable.

- Appropriate Gear: Equipping yourself with the right gear is essential for comfort and safety. A high-quality, well-fitted wetsuit acts as your first defence against the cold, enabling longer and more frequent immersions. Accessories like open water swim gloves, hydro booties or swim socks, and a neoprene cap can protect your extremities and head, which are most susceptible to heat loss. Additionally, investing in a changing mat, warm layers for post-swim recovery, and a sturdy kit bag will make your outings more practical and enjoyable.

The gear you choose may vary depending on the season. Commencing your cold-water journey in the warmer months, as I recommend, might seem inviting enough to forego heavier wetsuits or thermal layers. However, even during these milder conditions, the water can remain shockingly cold. Proper gear remains crucial to ensure you can comfortably adapt as the seasons change and as you push the boundaries of colder conditions.

For those fortunate enough to have access to organized lake facilities that cater specifically to cold-water swimmers, these venues often provide valuable resources such as daily water temperature reports and safety monitoring. These facilities are excellent for beginners as they offer a controlled environment to develop confidence and skill in cold-water swimming.

The following guide is crafted to accompany you through the stages of adapting to cold water. It offers insights and advice that progress with you, helping you to navigate the challenges and celebrate the milestones of your cold-water swimming adventure. Remember, preparation and prudence are your best allies in the quest to embrace and master the icy depths. Through careful planning, the right gear, and a supportive community, you can transform the daunting into the exhilarating.

General Guide on Water Temperatures & What to Expect

In the bone-chilling waters of 0-6°C (32-42.8°F), lovingly termed the "Baltic," each immersion is a trial by water. The initial shock sends a piercing chill straight to the bone, making even seasoned swimmers gasp for air as if an icy collar tightens around their neck. Skin prickles painfully upon contact, the acute cold rapidly depleting strength from every limb, transforming even a brief 25-meter swim into an epic feat. Emerging from these icy depths, lighter-skinned swimmers might notice their skin painted in stark shades of purple, orange, or red—striking proof of winter swimming's harsh embrace.

However, within this harsh environment lies a strange charm—an almost addictive cold water high. The surge of endorphins, the sheer thrill of overcoming nature's frosty barrier, acts as a powerful lure, drawing swimmers back into the frigid waters despite the discomfort. It's a compelling, yet challenging pursuit reserved for the brave, the seasoned and the most experienced – do not try this as a beginner!

As the temperature rises slightly to 6-11°C (42.8-51.8°F), a range fittingly called "Freezing," the initial pain and breathlessness mellow a little, offering just enough relief for the bold to venture further. Still perilous, these waters demand respect and expertise from those who choose to navigate their chilling currents.

The transition to 12-16°C (53.6-60.8°F) brings a milder setting known as "Fresh." This zone beckons triathletes and open-water enthusiasts who, clad in wetsuits, embrace the still-brisk waters. The challenges of the Baltic and Freezing zones transform here into a playground for the daring—a place where the thrill of the chill continues to entice.

With temperatures warming to a more comfortable 17-20°C (62.6-68°F), the season morphs into what's popularly celebrated as "Summer Swimming." Lakes and rivers transform into serene retreats, where sunseekers and families gather for leisurely swims and picnics by the water. The gentler conditions allow newcomers to acclimate to cold-water swimming in a more forgiving environment, making it a popular entry point for many.

As the mercury climbs above 21°C (69.8°F), the waters earn the label "Warm." Here, in the soothing lap of river pools and shallow lakes, swimmers find the freedom to linger indefinitely, revelling in long, unhindered swims. While the cool thrill of colder waters might be missed, this warmth provides a luxurious swimming experience that invites endless enjoyment and relaxation—a stark contrast to the rigorous demands of colder swims. This progression through temperatures forms a full spectrum of experiences, each with its own unique allure and challenge, captivating those who seek both the thrill of the cold and the comfort of the warm.

Making Plans: Find Water, Set a Schedule

Embarking on a journey into the invigorating world of cold-water swimming requires thoughtful planning and a strong commitment. To successfully kickstart your cold-water adventure, consider these detailed steps for a structured and enjoyable experience:

1. Set a Fixed Schedule: Develop a cold-water swim plan with a series of six scheduled swims. Choose a consistent time and location, ideally with a companion or group to keep motivation high and ensure safety. This regularity helps eliminate procrastination and last-minute cancellations. Complement your swim sessions with

a warm reward—perhaps a steaming cup of tea or coffee—to celebrate your resilience.

2. Choose Your Water Source Wisely: Natural bodies of water typically offer the best experience. If accessible, the ocean can provide varying temperatures and conditions which are ideal for adaptation. Alternatively, lakes, ponds, and gentle rivers are excellent choices, especially those designated for public swimming, as they often have monitored water quality and established access points which ensure safety.

3. Consistency is Key: Aim to swim at least once a week to foster and maintain the physiological adaptations to cold water. Infrequent swimming can diminish these benefits, making each swim feel like starting over. Over time, regular exposure will make the cold less daunting and more invigorating.

4. Start in Summer: Initiate your cold-water swimming in summer when temperatures are around 20°C (68°F). This warmer start helps ease the shock of cold water, allowing your body to adjust gradually as temperatures drop with the changing seasons. This approach is particularly beneficial for acclimatizing to colder conditions later in the year.

5. Choose the Right Time of Day: Tailor your swimming schedule to fit your daily routine and personal preference. Swimming in the late afternoon or early evening can feel warmer due to the sun heating the upper layers of water throughout the day. Additional-

ly, these times usually offer more daylight and potentially, a chance to swim under the setting sun, enhancing your experience with scenic beauty.

6. Equip Yourself Properly: Invest in quality swim gear suited for cold waters. A well-fitted wetsuit, neoprene gloves, and booties can significantly increase comfort and safety. These items not only provide insulation but also buoyancy and protection from natural elements.

7. Stay Informed and Prepared: Always check the weather and water conditions before each swim. Understanding the environment you're entering is crucial for safety. Additionally, bring along emergency contact information and basic first aid supplies in case of unexpected situations.

8. Join a Community: Becoming part of a local cold-water swimming group. These communities offer support, shared knowledge, and the camaraderie of like-minded enthusiasts. Plus, group settings can provide a sense of security for those new to cold-water swimming.

By carefully planning and following these guidelines, you'll not only ensure a safer cold-water swimming experience but also maximize the enjoyment and health benefits it brings. Remember, each swim is a step towards becoming more adept at navigating the challenges of cold-water immersion. Embrace the journey with enthusiasm and respect for the natural elements.

After emerging from the invigorating yet shocking embrace of cold waters, your body faces a critical challenge: recovering warmth safely and effectively. The process of re-warming is essential not just for comfort but to prevent the dangerous phenomenon known as "after drop," where your core temperature continues to fall even after exiting the water. To guide you through a safe recovery, consider the following detailed steps:

1. Dress Immediately: Begin by immediately removing any wet clothing. It's crucial to get dry as quickly as possible to stop further heat loss. Start with the upper body, which is key to heat retention, and work your way down. Use a dry, absorbent towel to pat yourself off, ensuring you're as dry as possible before dressing.

2. Layer Up: After drying, layer on clothing that will insulate and warm you efficiently. Begin with a thermal base layer to hold warmth close to your body. Add a fleece or wool sweater for mid-layer insulation and top it off with a windproof and waterproof jacket. Don't forget a woolly hat and gloves, as a significant amount of body heat escapes through the head and hands. In this scenario, unlike in running, swimmers do not generate excess heat post-exercise, rendering materials like silver foil blankets less effective.

3. Protect Your Feet: Cold feet can exacerbate the feeling of overall chill. While changing, stand on an insulating mat such as a changing mat or even a wooden board. Some experienced winter swimmers recommend standing in a shallow tub of warm water

poured from a thermos to quickly restore warmth to your feet.

4. Sip Warm Drinks: Internally warming your body with a hot beverage can help prevent the chill from settling in. Take a warm, soothing drink like herbal tea or a broth that can gently raise your internal temperature without shocking your system.

5. Refuel with Food: Eating a small, sugary snack can help quickly elevate your body temperature as your body metabolizes the food. This is particularly effective for swimmers who aren't showing signs of hypothermia, as quick sugars can spike energy levels and heat.

6. Seek Warmth: Move to a pre-warmed environment as soon as possible. This could be a heated car or a nearby building. Keeping the heat on can create a small oasis of warmth, aiding in your body's re-warming process.

7. Keep Moving: If you feel stable, engage in gentle physical activity to generate body heat. Simple movements like walking or lightly stretching can help stimulate circulation and warm you gradually.

8. Rest If Necessary: Listen to your body. If you begin to feel dizzy, nauseous, or unusually tired, take it as a sign to rest. Sit or lie down in a warm area, conserving energy and allowing your body to recover.

9. Be Cautious with Hot Baths and Showers: While a hot bath might seem like the perfect remedy, it can be dangerous for someone

who is very cold. The rapid change in temperature can cause blood vessels to dilate quickly, leading to a drop in blood pressure, which might make you feel faint or worse. If you choose this method, ensure the water is warm but not hot, and limit your time in the water.

By implementing these steps, you can ensure a safe and comfortable transition back to warmth after a cold-water swim. Prioritizing your warmth and overall well-being is essential for reaping the invigorating benefits of cold-water swimming safely and enjoyably.

· • • ● • ● • • ·

Practical Lessons from Getting Started – Preparing for the Cold Water:

Acclimatization Process:

- Initial dives are marked by intense cold and fear, counterbalanced by excitement and the thrill of the unknown.

- Subsequent swims involve overcoming the heightened sensation of cold as novelty fades, transitioning into a profound mental and physical engagement with the environment.

- Acclimatization to cold water is gradual, requiring persistence and regular exposure, typically recommended as at least six dips.

- Each swim builds endurance, enhances cold tolerance, and deepens the swimmer's connection with this extreme activity.

Basic Requirements and Precautions:

- Cold-water swimming is fundamentally simple but requires knowing how to swim and involves extensive preparation and precaution to ensure safety.

- Essential considerations include choosing a safe and suitable location, swimming with a companion for safety, and wearing appropriate gear to protect against the cold.

Practical Preparations:

- Select a location that aligns with your swimming ability and environmental conditions, ensuring it's safe and accessible.

- Always swim with a partner to enhance safety and enjoyment, and to aid in case of emergency.

- Equip with proper gear like a high-quality wetsuit, thermal layers, and protective accessories to maintain body heat and mobility.

Seasonal Considerations and Facilities:

- Start cold-water swimming in warmer months to gradually adapt to the cold as seasons change.

- Utilize facilities like organized lake systems that provide safety features, temperature monitoring, and controlled environments ideal for beginners.

Comprehensive Guide and Support:

- The journey in cold-water swimming is supported by a guide that offers insights and advice tailored to different stages of adaptation, emphasizing preparation and safety.

- Engage with a community or group for shared experiences, increased motivation, and additional security.

By adhering to these guidelines, swimmers can safely explore the exhilarating world of cold-water swimming, turning daunting initial experiences into enjoyable and invigorating activities.

Chapter Six

The Benefits of Cold-Water Swimming for Women

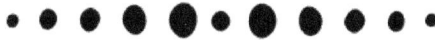

• • • ● • ● • • •

Ease Menopause & Other Menstrual Symptoms

Within this chapter, we delve into recent research that review the profound benefits of cold-water swimming specifically tailored to women in relation to symptoms associated with the menopause and other menstrual symptoms. This therapeutic practice offers promising support for managing various symptoms associated with menstruation and the transitional phases leading up to menopause.

Menstruation, a natural biological process, often carries with it a spectrum of physical and emotional challenges that can significantly impact a woman's overall quality of life and well-being. Beyond the mere act of bleeding, menstruation encompasses a wide array of symptoms that can vary widely among individuals. These symptoms may include premenstrual syndrome (PMS), characterized by mood swings, anxiety, depression, and fatigue, as well as menstrual cramps (dysmenorrhea), breast tenderness, bloating, headaches, food cravings, digestive issues, acne, and skin changes [1]. These symptoms are primarily driven by fluctuations in the sex hormones oestrogen and progesterone, although it's important to acknowledge that menstrual experiences can differ greatly.

For many women, the journey through menstruation is marked by a complex interplay of physical discomfort and emotional turbulence. These experiences often extend beyond the menstrual cycle itself, shaping women's perceptions and management of their reproductive health throughout their lives. However, emerging research suggests that cold-water swimming may offer a holistic approach to alleviate these burdensome symptoms and promote overall well-being.

By exploring the therapeutic potential of cold-water swimming tailored to women's unique physiological and psychological needs, we aim to shed light on a promising avenue for enhancing women's health and to embrace the menstrual cycles and menopausal transitions with greater resilience and vitality.

As a woman approaches the end of her reproductive years, she enters a stage known as perimenopause. This pivotal period, characterized by fluctuating hormone levels, heralds the onset of menopause, officially defined as the absence of menstruation for 12 consecutive months, thereby marking the transition to the postmenopausal stage. The perimenopausal journey typically spans approximately four years, though this timeline can vary from individual to individual [2].

During perimenopause, women may encounter a host of symptoms reminiscent of those experienced during menstruation, including mood swings, hot flushes, and hormonal fluctuations. These symptoms, coupled with the uncertainty and physical changes inherent in the transition, can significantly impact a woman's overall quality of life during this phase. Managing these perimenopausal symptoms is paramount, as they have the potential to disrupt daily activities, strain relationships, and compromise emotional well-being. By implementing effective coping strategies and embracing supportive interventions such as cold-water swimming, women navigating perimenopause can cultivate resilience and regain a sense of control over their health and vitality.

In the pages that follow, we delve deeper into the therapeutic benefits of cold-water swimming for women during perimenopause, exploring how this immersive experience can provide relief from symptoms, promote hormonal balance, and foster a sense of empowerment and rejuvenation during this transformative phase of life.

The Cooling Relief of Cold-Water

Recent research has highlighted an unconventional yet promising approach to managing menstrual and perimenopausal symptom through cold water swimming [3]. This comprehensive study led by distinguished researchers from the Elizabeth Garrett Anderson Institute for Women's Health at University College London explored the effects of cold-water immersion on these symptoms and whilst this is just one single piece of research, the findings offer hope to women who are suffering.

The ground-breaking study enlisted a diverse cohort of 1,114 women spanning a wide age range from 16 to 80 years old, with an average age of 49. Notably, a significant portion of the participants, comprising 785 women, were traversing the often-challenging phase of menopause. Amidst the fluctuating hormonal landscape and the accompanying array of symptoms, these women discovered solace and relief within the invigorating embrace of cold-water immersion.

The findings of the study revealed remarkable outcomes, with half of the menopausal participants reporting a profound reduction in anxiety levels after engaging in cold water swimming. Beyond anxiety relief, the therapeutic benefits extended to other aspects of well-being, with 35% experiencing decreased mood swings, 31% reporting alleviation of low mood, and 30% noting a reduction in the frequency and intensity of hot flushes.

Perhaps most striking was the resounding consensus among the participants, with a resounding 63% actively seeking out cold water swimming as a targeted intervention to manage their menopausal symptoms. This widespread adoption underscores the activity's remarkable effectiveness in addressing the multifaceted challenges of menopause, offering a beacon of hope and empowerment to women navigating this transformative phase of life.

As we delve deeper into the implications of these findings, it becomes increasingly evident that cold water swimming holds immense promise as a holistic and accessible therapeutic modality for women during menopause.

By shedding light on the nuanced interplay between cold water immersion and menopausal symptom management, this can be used as a tool that women can use to help with this natural transition.

Personal Stories of Transformation

The personal narratives shared by the study participants offer poignant insights into the transformative power of cold-water swimming, imbuing the data with a rich, human element. One participant, a 54-year-old woman, articulated the profound impact of cold-water swimming on her menopausal journey, remarking:

> 'Cold-water swimming has had a profound effect on my menopausal symptoms. Exercising amidst nature, whether in solitary contemplation or in the company of fellow women, feels inherently healing.' [3]

Her testimony not only underscores the therapeutic benefits of cold-water immersion but also highlights the importance of connection and camaraderie in fostering resilience and well-being.

Similarly, a 57-year-old participant shared a compelling testament to the transformative potential of cold-water immersion, proclaiming:

'Cold water is phenomenal. It has saved my life. In the water, I feel invincible. All symptoms, both physical and mental, dissipate, and I rediscover my true essence.'

Her words echo the sentiment of many, revealing the profound sense of liberation and empowerment that cold water swimming can instil, transcending mere symptom relief to awaken a deeper sense of self and vitality.

Amidst the wealth of personal anecdotes, five overarching themes emerged from the participants' open-ended responses, encapsulating the multifaceted benefits of cold-water swimming:

1. The Calming and Mood-Boosting Effect of Water: Many participants attested to the soothing and uplifting influence of cold-water immersion, describing a profound sense of calm and clarity that envelops them during and after their swims.

2. Companionship and Community: The communal aspect of cold-water swimming emerged as a recurring theme, with participants highlighting the invaluable support, camaraderie, and shared laughter that accompany these gatherings, fostering a sense of belonging and solidarity.

3. Period Improvements: Several women noted improvements in menstrual symptoms, including reduced cramping, bloating, and discomfort, suggesting that cold water swimming may offer holistic relief for menstrual-related challenges.

4. Relief from Hot Flushes: Many menopausal participants reported a significant reduction in the frequency and intensity of hot flushes, attributing this relief to the cooling effects of cold-water immersion on their bodies.

5. Overall, Health Improvement: Beyond specific symptoms, participants spoke of a holistic improvement in their overall health and well-being, citing increased energy, resilience, and vitality as tangible benefits of their cold-water swimming regimen.

Scientific and Cultural Significance

The research not only sheds light on the physical and mental health benefits of cold-water swimming but also underscores its profound social implications. Professor Joyce Harper, the study's senior author, underscored the anecdotal evidence supporting the practice's ability to alleviate physical symptoms such as hot flushes, aches, and pains.

Moreover, the study revealed that the duration of swimming and the temperature of the water played pivotal roles in determining the extent of the benefits experienced. Among the 711 women who reported menstrual symptoms, a staggering 38% reported better control over mood swings after engaging in cold water swimming. This promising finding highlights the broader applicability of cold-water swimming in managing symptoms across different stages of women's reproductive health, from menstruation to menopause and beyond.

Other studies exploring the potential benefits of cold-water swimming, particularly in the context of pregnant women's health, suggest intriguing possibilities as to the mechanistic processes that may be responsible for these benefits [4]. Research indicates that regular cold-water swimming may have the potential to reduce stress levels, offering a pathway to improved obstetric outcomes. The underlying hypothesis suggests that cold water swimming serves as a significant physiological stressor, which, upon habitual exposure, could potentially modulate the body's stress response, leading to positive health outcomes.

Central to this hypothesis is the burgeoning popularity of cold-water swimming, fuelled by its widely advertised benefits, including mood enhancement and stress reduction [5]. While anecdotal evidence abounds, there remains a pressing need for rigorous scientific inquiry to discern between correlation and causation regarding the purported health benefits associated with cold water immersion. While the hypothesis presents compelling possibilities, it underscores the necessity for further empirical research to substantiate these claims and elucidate the underlying mechanisms at play.

Moreover, ongoing investigation is essential to delineate the specific variables that may optimize symptom relief for menopausal and menstrual conditions. This includes exploring factors such as the frequency, duration, temperature, and extent of cold-water exposure necessary to elicit therapeutic benefits. By delving deeper into these nuanced variables, researchers can refine existing hypotheses and develop targeted interventions tailored to women's unique reproductive health needs.

In summary the research reflects a significant shift towards natural and holistic approaches in healthcare, particularly for women's health issues. Cold water swimming emerges not just as a physical activity but as a multifaceted therapy that offers psychological relief, community building, and a deep, invigorating connection to nature. Whilst the research is based on the perception of women, via an extensive survey, it becomes increasingly clear that cold water swimming represents not only a therapeutic modality for individual well-being but also a catalyst for social change. By offering a holistic approach to managing physical and emotional symptoms, cold water swimming has the potential to empower women to reclaim agency over their health and embrace active, vibrant lifestyles. As we strive to foster a culture of inclusivity and empowerment in the realm of women's health, cold water swimming emerges as a beacon of hope, resilience, and transformation.

• • • ● ● • ● ● • • •

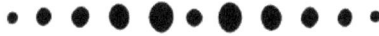

Practical Lessons from The Benefits of Cold-Water Swimming for Women:

- **Cold-Water Swimming for Women's Health**: Recent research explores the profound benefits of cold-water swimming tailored specifically to women, offering promising support for managing menstrual and perimenopausal symptoms.

- **Menstrual Challenges and Cold-Water Swimming**: Menstruation brings physical and emotional challenges, including PMS, mood swings, and discomfort. Cold-water swimming may offer a holistic approach to alleviate these symptoms and promote overall well-being.

- **Perimenopause and Cold-Water Swimming**: Perimenopause, marked by hormonal fluctuations, can be accompanied by symptoms like mood swings and hot flushes. Cold-water swimming may provide relief and empowerment during this transitional phase.

- **Study Findings**: A comprehensive study involving 1,114 women revealed significant benefits of cold-water swimming, including reduced anxiety, mood swings, low mood, and hot flushes among menopausal participants.

- **Personal Testimonies**: Personal stories from participants underscore the transformative power of cold-water swimming, emphasizing its calming effect, community aspect, and relief from menstrual and menopausal symptoms.

- **Themes from Participant Responses**: Five main themes emerged from participant responses, including the calming effect of water, companionship, period improvements, relief from hot flushes, and overall health improvement.

- **Scientific and Cultural Significance**: The research highlights not only the physical and mental health benefits but also the social implications of cold-water swimming. Further scientific inquiry is needed to understand its mechanisms and optimize symptom relief.

- **Shift Towards Holistic Approaches**: Cold water swimming represents a shift towards natural and holistic approaches in women's healthcare, offering psychological relief, community building, and a deep connection to nature.

Chapter Seven

Cryotherapy & Contrast Therapy

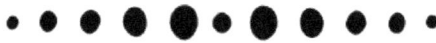

• • • ● • ● ● • • •

Recover Faster, Better Manage Pain & Improved Mood

B y delving into the scientific research surrounding cryotherapy and contrast therapy, we explore how these traditional methods can be enhanced through contemporary scientific insights to significantly boost recovery from injuries and enhance our mood and overall well-being. Cryotherapy, which employs extreme cold to reduce pain and swelling, works in tandem with contrast therapy, a technique that alternates between hot and cold temperatures. This combination yields a synergistic effect that can greatly improve health outcomes and recovery times. We will explore the mechanisms behind these therapies and provide practical guidance on how to integrate them into your daily routine for optimal health benefits.

The Essence of the Cold: Cryotherapy

Cryotherapy, broadly defined, encompasses a variety of therapeutic techniques that harness the power of cold temperatures. Its primary objective is to extract heat by lowering core and tissue temperatures and altering blood flow. The efficacy of cryotherapy stems chiefly from its ability to decelerate sensory nerves, thereby yielding significant health benefits. Its historical application in managing both primary and secondary tissue injuries and associated inflammations is well-documented [1]. Additionally, the traditional Finnish regimen of alternating between sauna sessions and cold plunges—a practice known as contrast therapy—illustrates an age-old technique that merges the therapeutic effects of both heat and cold. This method is purported to confer a range of health benefits, including a potential increase in lifespan. Although further research is necessary to fully verify this claim, this book delves into the existing studies that support the broad spectrum of health benefits cryotherapy can offer, discussing research-backed methods to safely integrate these practices into everyday life.

The Physiological Impact of Cold

There are various ways to experience cold stress, ranging from plunging into an ice bath, taking a brisk cold shower, and in the extreme, stepping into a cryotherapy chamber. Like heat stress, cold stress acts as a type of hormetic stress. This stress activates genetic pathways that enhance our resilience and capability to handle stress in everyday life. Specifically, cold exposure leads to increases in norepinephrine within the locus coeruleus region of the brain, a key area involved in regulating focus, attention, vigilance, and mood. Although norepinephrine is pharmacologically used to treat conditions such as depression and attention deficit hyperactivity disorder (ADHD), it can also be naturally stimulated by cold-induced shocks to the body.

Exposure to 14°C (57.2°F) for 30 minutes can boost plasma norepinephrine concentration levels by 530% compared with baseline.[2]

It is crucial to understand that the colder the water, the less time it takes to stimulate the release of norepinephrine, a key hormone in the body's stress response. However, colder temperatures also heighten the risk of hypothermia, making caution imperative when engaging with extremely cold environments.

A prudent approach to safely experience cold exposure is to begin with a conventional warm shower and incrementally adjust the temperature towards cooler settings until it becomes slightly uncomfortable. Gradually introducing cold water over a span of days and weeks allows the body to adapt progressively, reducing the risk of shock. This method is particularly beneficial as it minimizes potential dangers for individuals with specific health vulnerabilities. By carefully moderating the exposure to cold, it is possible to harness its benefits while safeguarding health.

Exploring further into the physiological nuances, cryotherapy offers a compelling illustration of how temperature manipulation can confer significant health benefits. By lowering the temperature of body tissues, cryotherapy not only reduces the transmission of pain signals through sensory nerves, offering a natural, non-invasive form of pain relief, but also plays a vital role in managing the body's inflammatory response to both primary and secondary tissue damage.

In essence, cryotherapy—with its profound historical significance and physiological impacts—stands as a pillar of therapeutic practices. By embracing the therapeutic use of cold, we tap into an ancient reservoir of healing that not only provides relief and aids recovery but also connects us to a longstanding tradition of health optimization. As we continue to delve into and validate the benefits of cryotherapy and temperature contrast therapies, we pave new avenues toward wellness, rooted in the ancient wisdom of our ancestors yet enhanced by the advancements of modern science.

Cold Therapy

In sports, at all competitive levels, applying ice is a prevalent method for managing injuries, particularly for sprains. The primary purpose of this practice is to control internal swelling without compromising joint mobility. Beyond reducing swelling, ice is also effective for pain management, functioning without the need for painkillers or other medications. It alleviates pain by temporarily decelerating the speed of nerve signals, thus lessening the intensity of pain. Moreover, the sensation of cold shifts your focus away from the pain. Ice application also induces vasoconstriction, where blood vessels supplying the injured area constrict, reducing both swelling and inflammation.

For those suffering from inflammatory injuries, incorporating ice into the treatment regimen is advisable, along with seeking professional medical guidance. It is most effective to apply ice immediately following the injury for no more than 20 minutes at a time. This can be repeated every two to three hours during the first 12 hours post-injury. Caution is advised to avoid placing ice directly on the skin, as it can cause burns. Protect the skin by placing a barrier, such as a cloth or even a bag of frozen peas, between the ice and your skin. This simple measure ensures effective treatment while preventing skin damage.

A Cautionary Note if Weightlifting

Cold compressions and immersions are frequently utilized between exercise sessions to facilitate recovery. Yet, their impact on strength training remains somewhat ambiguous. Recent studies, such as one conducted by Peake et al. in 2020, indicate that cold water immersion might negate some of the benefits associated with strength training. This adverse effect is believed to stem from the cold's suppression of gene and protein expression critical for muscle growth pathways. [3]

For those concerned about these potential drawbacks, adjusting the timing of cold exposures could prove beneficial. Consider engaging in a cold shower or bath several hours post-weight training sessions, or alternatively, time your cold exposures either before your workouts or on days you do not train. This strategy allows you to reap the rejuvenating and energizing advantages of cold immersion without undermining your strength training progress.

Contrast Therapy

Alternating between cold and heat, known as contrast therapy, can offer significant benefits for treating common joint and muscle-related ailments. This type of immersion therapy does not require extreme temperatures. For instance, "hot" can refer to temperatures ranging from 38°C (100.4°F) to 48°C (118.4°F), while "cold" encompasses a more moderate range from 10°C (50°F) to 18°C (64.4°F). Research, including studies on conditions like osteoporosis, suggests that contrast therapy can be beneficial, although more investigation is needed to fully understand the physiological mechanisms involved.

A seminal study by Myrer, Draper, and Durrant in 1994 highlights that the alternating expansion and contraction of blood vessels during contrast therapy act like a pump [4]. This process enhances oxygen delivery to muscle tissues and facilitates the removal of waste products, both crucial for aiding recovery.

- Increase oxygenation to muscles

- Enhance waste removal through pumping waste on blood vessels

- Support overall recovery

These findings underscore the potential of contrast therapy as a simple yet effective treatment modality for enhancing muscular health and recovery.

A Method to Reduce Stress Levels

Contrast therapy offers benefits beyond muscle recovery. A notable study involving young men demonstrated significant health improvements following a regimen of four cycles, each consisting of 12 minutes in a sauna followed by one minute of cold-water immersion. Remarkably, this routine led to an almost 30% reduction in the stress hormone cortisol. Additionally, this hot/cold cycling not only reduced stress but also boosted energy levels and surprisingly decreased the amount of sick leave taken, as reported in a randomized controlled trial involving 3,000 volunteers [5]. Participants who experienced these benefits, reported such dramatic improvements in their overall health and energy that many continued with contrast therapy beyond the study. This approach has been found to be quite accessible; for instance, a 30-second shower has been shown to be just as effective as one lasting 90 seconds. Moreover, similar benefits can be achieved by gradually adjusting the water temperature from warm to cold. While these findings are encouraging, it's crucial to consult with a healthcare provider before starting contrast therapy, especially for those with or recovering from heart conditions, as the initial temperature shock can temporarily increase blood pressure. This therapy offers a promising, simple method to enhance well-being and reduce stress, making it a valuable tip for anyone looking to improve their health regime.

• • • ● • ● ● • •

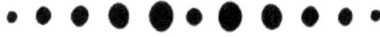

Practical Lessons from Cryotherapy & Contrast Therapy:

- **Harnessing the Cold:** Cold therapy can significantly reduce swelling, alleviate pain, and facilitate recovery following an injury. This simple, effective approach can be a key component in your post-injury care regimen.

- **Balancing Heat with Cold:** Alternating between heat and cold not only enhances mood and energy levels but also can lead to fewer sick days. This contrast therapy taps into the body's natural healing mechanisms, promoting overall well-being.

- **Incorporating Contrast Showers:** A straightforward method to introduce the benefits of contrast therapy into your daily routine is through showers. Starting with a hot shower and then switching to cold can invigorate your body, improving circulation and boosting energy. This simple practice is a convenient way to experience the therapeutic effects of temperature variation.

Chapter Eight

Embracing Seasonal Changes for Better Sleep

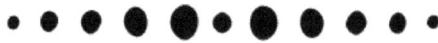

• • • ● • ● • • •

Adapting Your Routine for Restful Nights

As many of us experience, the winter months bring longer nights and shorter days, often nudging us to retire to bed earlier. This change in daylight can also make waking up in the morning more challenging due to the reduced exposure to natural light. Interestingly, sleep tracking technology has revealed that during these winter months, not only do we tend to sleep longer, but the quality of our sleep also improves significantly. Many of us experience extended periods of deep sleep, which is crucial for physical and mental restoration.

Understanding Different States of Sleep

Sleep, contrary to common belief, is not a passive state but a dynamic process vital for our well-being. Sleep experts categorize sleep into two main types: Rapid Eye Movement (REM) and Non-Rapid Eye Movement (NREM) sleep. Each type is crucial for various aspects of health and cognitive function.

NREM Sleep: Three States:

- Stage 1: The transition from wakefulness to sleep.

- Stage 2: Light sleep, during which body temperature drops and heart rate slows.

- Stage 3: Deep sleep, essential for physical recovery and growth hormone release.

REM Sleep: Occurring roughly 90 minutes after falling asleep, this stage is characterized by rapid eye movements, increased brain activity, and vivid dreams. It plays a critical role in memory consolidation and emotional regulation.

Throughout a typical night, you will cycle through these stages' multiple times. The architecture of these cycles changes as the night progresses, with more NREM sleep occurring in the first half of the night and an increase in REM sleep towards the morning. Most people spend approximately 75% to 80% of their total sleep time in NREM sleep.

The Role of Light in Sleep Quality

The absence of natural light in winter can significantly impact our sleep-wake cycle, also known as the circadian rhythm. This rhythm is influenced by the environmental light-dark cycle and dictates when we feel alert and when we feel sleepy. In winter, the extended darkness can lead to increased melatonin production, a hormone that promotes sleep, thus explaining why we may feel sleepier and find it easier to sleep longer.

Enhancing Sleep in Winter

To mitigate the challenges of waking up on dark winter mornings, consider using a light therapy lamp to simulate sunrise. This can help adjust your circadian rhythm by reducing melatonin production at the right time, making it easier to wake up. Additionally, maintaining a consistent sleep schedule, even on weekends, can help stabilize your sleep patterns and improve sleep quality over time.

The Significance of Sleep Stages

Understanding the significance of different sleep stages and how they contribute to brain health and physical well-being underscores the importance of getting a balanced cycle of REM and NREM sleep. While REM sleep helps with emotional and cognitive processes, NREM sleep is indispensable for physical health and recovery. Therefore, appreciating the complexity of sleep can motivate better sleep habits and, subsequently, better health.

The Impact of NREM Sleep on Health and Disease

Non-Rapid Eye Movement (NREM) sleep is essential not only for physical recovery but also for cognitive function, particularly memory consolidation. Recent studies have highlighted potential links between abnormalities in NREM sleep processes and several neurological disorders. For instance, disruptions in NREM sleep have been implicated in the pathology of diseases such as Schizophrenia, Epilepsy, Alzheimer's, and Parkinson's disease [1], [2], [3], [4], [5]. These findings suggest that the quality and quantity of NREM sleep may have far-reaching implications for neurodegenerative and psychiatric conditions.

NREM Sleep and Cardiovascular Health

NREM sleep, particularly during slow wave sleep—the deepest stage of sleep—plays a protective role in cardiovascular health. During this stage, blood pressure significantly drops, which can help reduce the risk of heart disease. However, individuals suffering from sleep apnoea, chronic insomnia, or high blood pressure, or those who experience frequently interrupted sleep, often do not experience this beneficial drop in blood pressure. This absence can elevate their risk of developing cardiovascular problems.

The Influence of Body Temperature on Sleep and Health

One less appreciated aspect of our sleep cycle is how our body temperature interacts with it. Typically, as night approaches, our core body temperature decreases by about 1°C (33.8°F), signalling that it's time to sleep. This reduction helps trigger the circadian rhythm, syncing our internal clock with environmental cues. However, when this drop in core temperature doesn't align with an individual's sleep schedule—such as in the case of shift workers or those with irregular sleeping habits—it can lead to significant health issues. These groups are at an elevated risk for conditions like heart disease and type 2 diabetes [6].

Furthermore, a lower core temperature at night not only signals the body to prepare for sleep but also enhances sleep quality. Failing to sleep during this natural dip can lead to reduced alertness and slower reaction times during the day. This is particularly relevant for those who work at night or have altered sleep cycles due to lifestyle or occupational demands.

A key to enhancing sleep quality and overall health is synchronizing sleep patterns with the body's natural temperature rhythms. Here are detailed strategies to help you achieve this alignment:

Maintain a Regular Sleep Schedule

Consistency is crucial for stabilizing your circadian rhythm. Aim to go to bed and wake up at the same time every day, even on weekends. This regularity helps your body anticipate when to initiate sleep processes, making it easier to fall asleep and wake up naturally.

Create a Pre-Sleep Routine

Developing a calming pre-sleep routine can significantly improve your ability to fall asleep. Consider these activities:

- Engage in Light Reading: Choose light, non-stimulating materials to help your mind unwind.

- Take a Warm Bath or Visit a Sauna: Though initially warming, your body's subsequent natural cooling process after these activities can promote faster sleep onset.

- Practice Relaxation Techniques: Activities such as yoga, meditation, or deep-breathing exercises can reduce stress and prepare your body for sleep.

Optimize Your Sleeping Environment

The environment in which you sleep can profoundly affect sleep quality. Optimal conditions include:

- Cool Temperature: Set your bedroom temperature around 18°C (64°F) to support the body's natural dip in temperature.

- Reduce Noise and Light: Use blackout curtains and consider white noise machines to create an ideal sleeping atmosphere.

- Comfortable Bedding: Invest in high-quality mattresses and pillows that support your body and enhance comfort.

Consider Light Exposure

Light exposure has a powerful effect on your circadian rhythm:

- Maximize Daylight Exposure: Try to get natural sunlight exposure, especially in the morning. This signals your brain to wake up and helps regulate sleep patterns.

- Limit Evening Light: Reduce exposure to blue light from screens and artificial lights in the evening. Consider using devices with night modes or blue light filters in the hours leading up to bed-time.

Adapt Your Diet for Better Sleep

What you eat and when you eat can also influence your sleep:

- Avoid Large Meals and Caffeine Before Bed: Eating a heavy meal or consuming caffeine close to bedtime can disrupt your sleep. Try to have your last big meal at least 3-4 hours before you go to sleep.

- Consider Sleep-Promoting Snacks: Foods containing tryptophan, magnesium, and calcium can promote sleep. A small snack of yogurt, bananas, or wholegrain crackers can be beneficial.

Address Psychological Factors

Often overlooked, psychological stressors can disrupt your natural sleep rhythm:

- Manage Stress: Regular exercise and mindfulness practices can reduce stress levels, making it easier to sleep.

- Seek Professional Help if Needed: Persistent sleep disturbances might be a sign of underlying issues such as anxiety or insomnia. Consulting a healthcare provider can provide tailored strategies and treatments.

Implementing these strategies not only helps synchronize your sleep patterns with natural rhythms but also improves the duration and quality of your sleep, leading to better health and well-being.

Optimize Your Sleeping Environment

Creating the ideal sleeping environment is crucial for enhancing sleep quality. A cool, dark environment is essential, but it's important to understand that 'cool' means pleasantly cool, not uncomfortably cold. Let's explore the science behind this and practical ways to achieve the optimal sleeping conditions.

The Science of Cool Sleep Environments

Research consistently shows that cooler room temperatures can significantly improve the quality of sleep by aligning with your body's internal biological clock that naturally cools down during the night. A key study into this found that volunteers sleeping in a room maintained at 17°C and 62.6°F experienced deeper sleep and spent a higher percentage of the night in stage 3 NREM sleep, the most restorative phase [7]. This stage is crucial for memory consolidation, brain health, tissue repair, and strengthening the immune system. Furthermore, cooler temperatures also promote increased REM sleep, the stage associated with dreaming, memory processing, and emotional regulation.

Practical Tips for Cooling Down Your Sleep

1. Use Air Flow to Your Advantage: Fans or Air Conditioning: These can help maintain a constant temperature throughout the night. Fans can also provide white noise that helps drown out disruptive sounds. Open Windows: If conditions allow, an open window can bring in fresh, cool air and improve air circulation, which is beneficial for both temperature control and air quality.

2. Optimal Temperature Range: The ideal temperature for sleep is between 16°C to 20°C and 60.8°F to 68°F respectively. This range helps facilitate the natural drop in body temperature that signals your brain it's time for sleep.

3. Adjust Based on Health and Age: The elderly and very young, or those with certain medical conditions, may require a slightly

warmer environment to avoid the risks associated with getting too cold.

Advanced Strategies for Managing Sleep Environment

1. Use Adaptive Bedding: Invest in breathable, moisture-wicking sheets and bedding that can help regulate body temperature throughout the night.

2. Smart Home Technology: Consider using smart thermostats that automatically adjust the room temperature according to present sleep and wake times.

3. Be Mindful of Humidity: Both high and low humidity levels can impact sleep quality. A humidifier or dehumidifier can help maintain an ideal humidity level, generally recommended between 40-60%.

A Case Study on Sleep Apnoea

A randomized controlled trial examined the influence of different room temperatures on individuals diagnosed with obstructive sleep apnoea, a sleep disorder characterized by temporary blockages of the airway. Participants in the study were assigned to sleep in environments maintained at three distinct temperatures: 16°C (60.8°F), 20°C (68°F), and 24°C (75.2°F). This segmentation aimed to determine how varying degrees of coolness affected sleep quality and overall alertness upon waking.

The outcomes indicated significant differences among the groups. Individuals in the coolest environment, 16°C (60.8°F), not only had longer sleep durations but also experienced fewer instances of wakefulness throughout the night. Additionally, they reported feeling more alert and refreshed the following morning. In contrast, those sleeping at 20°C (68°F) and 24°C (75.2°F) showed incremental decreases in sleep quality and alertness.

These findings emphasize the importance of optimal temperature settings in the bedrooms of individuals with sleep disorders. Regulating room temperature could be a straightforward, non-invasive approach to improve sleep quality and enhance daytime functioning for those affected by obstructive sleep apnoea. This study contributes to a growing body of evidence suggesting environmental factors, such as room temperature, play a crucial role in managing and potentially alleviating symptoms of sleep disorders.

How to Improve Your Sleep

To optimize sleep quality, it's crucial to maintain a cool, dark environment. Achieving the ideal coolness, which is distinct from cold, can be facilitated using a fan, air conditioning, or even better, by allowing fresh air through an open window. This not only keeps the air circulating but also helps maintain a cooler temperature conducive to sleep. Cooler room temperatures align with our internal biological clock, helping us fall asleep faster and achieve deeper sleep stages.

Delving into the scientific basis, cooler temperatures positively influence our core body temperature, which is pivotal for initiating and maintaining sleep. Research highlights that a lower core body temperature helps us fall asleep quicker and remain in deep sleep longer. For example, one study, healthy volunteers experienced enhanced sleep quality when their sleep environments were set to either 17°C (62.6°F) or 22°C (71.6°F) [8]. Participants in the cooler 17°C setting spent a greater portion of the night in NREM stage 3 sleep, which is crucial for memory consolidation, brain health, tissue repair, and strengthening the immune system. Additionally, sleeping in a cooler environment increased the time spent in REM sleep, essential for dreaming and processing emotions.

Further research in a randomized controlled trial involving 40 participants with obstructive sleep apnoea—a condition where the airway is blocked intermittently during sleep due to the tongue falling back—underscored the benefits of cooler sleep environments. Participants were divided into three groups, sleeping at temperatures of 16°C (60.8°F), 20°C (68°F), and 24°C (75.2°F). Those in the coolest environment of 16°C

(60.8°F), slept significantly longer, experienced less wakefulness, and were more alert upon waking.

For general guidance, maintaining a bedroom temperature between 16°C (60.8°F) and 20°C (68°F) is advisable, though care should be taken to avoid getting too cold, particularly for the elderly or very young. Adjusting room temperature can be as simple as opening a window to lower the temperature, depending on the season and your geographic location, while also improving ventilation. This straightforward adjustment can have profound benefits for sleep quality and overall health.

The Role of Heat Before Bed

If you find it difficult to fall asleep, consider engaging in relaxing activities such as taking a warm bath, shower, or enjoying a sauna session one to two hours before bedtime. These activities can effectively raise your body temperature temporarily, setting off a natural cooling process as you get closer to bedtime. This cooling aligns with your body's natural preparation for sleep, making it easier to fall asleep. Additionally, though it may lack aesthetic appeal, wearing socks to bed can warm your feet, leading to a slight drop in your core body temperature, further facilitating the onset of sleep. These methods are aimed at synchronizing your circadian rhythm with your body's inherent sleep-wake cycle, promoting a seamless transition into deep, rejuvenating sleep.

As the night progresses, your core body temperature naturally decreases, typically reaching its lowest point around 4 AM, usually a few hours before you wake. It then starts to rise in anticipation of the day ahead. Maintaining a cooler bedroom environment is crucial for enhancing overall sleep quality. While many prefer a warm sleeping environment, overly warm conditions can significantly disrupt sleep.

A study examining the effects of extreme weather on sleep, which analysed data from over 750,000 individuals across the USA, revealed a definitive correlation between sleep quality and unusual weather patterns [9]. The research found that high temperatures were linked to an increase in sleep disturbances. In contrast, cooler temperatures, even those below freezing, were shown to enhance sleep quality. This is not to advocate for sleeping in dangerously cold conditions due to the risk of hypothermia, but it underscores how lower temperatures can improve sleep efficiency, which may benefit neurological health over time.

The broader implications of these findings are increasingly pertinent in the context of global warming. Rising global temperatures, particularly during the night, pose a significant threat to sleep quality, affecting demographics such as women and individuals over the age of 65 disproportionately. Predictive models indicate that with the ongoing increase in global temperatures, we could be losing an average of 10 minutes of sleep nightly, totalling over 60 hours lost per year. This significant decrease emphasizes the urgent need for adaptive strategies to counteract the impact of warmer nights on our sleep patterns and overall health, ensuring better quality of life in a changing climate.

In summary, embrace the chill of cold nights and explore the significant benefits they offer for improving your sleep quality. Cooler temperatures naturally align with your body's circadian rhythms, promoting deeper and more restorative sleep. This adjustment in your sleeping environment can help lower your core body temperature, signalling to your body that it's time to wind down and rest, which facilitates a quicker transition to sleep and a longer duration of deep sleep.

Cold weather can also influence your sleep by enhancing the overall environment of your bedroom. Maintaining a cooler room temperature not only helps in reducing wakefulness throughout the night but also minimizes disruptions caused by overheating, which is often linked to poor sleep quality.

If taking a warm bath doesn't help you sleep, adopting the counter measure of cold adaptation may be for you, through methods like taking a cold shower before bed as this can reinforce your body's readiness for sleep by enhancing blood circulation and reducing stress. This can be particularly beneficial for those who have trouble falling asleep, as it helps calm the mind and prepare the body for rest.

Consider using the colder months as a strategic period to focus on and improve your sleep hygiene. This can involve adjusting your bedroom to cooler temperatures, adopting bedtime routines that incorporate elements of cold exposure, and ensuring your sleeping environment supports uninterrupted sleep. By optimizing these aspects, you can harness the natural benefits of cold to enhance your sleep, thereby improving your overall health and well-being.

Practical Lessons from Embracing Seasonal Changes for Better Sleep:

- **Light and Sleep Quality**: Reduced sunlight in winter increases melatonin production, enhancing sleepiness and extending sleep duration. Light therapy lamps can simulate sunrise to help adjust the circadian rhythm and ease waking up on dark mornings.

- **Enhancing Winter Sleep**: Maintain a consistent sleep schedule. Use a pre-sleep routine involving warm baths or relaxation techniques to induce the body's natural cooling mechanism, aiding sleep onset.

- **Significance of Sleep Stages**: Balanced cycles of REM and NREM sleep are vital for comprehensive health benefits, influencing everything from cognitive function to physical recovery.

- **Health Implications of NREM Sleep**: Critical for cognitive functions and linked to reduced risks of neurological and cardiovascular diseases.

- **Temperature's Role in Sleep**: A cooler bedroom environment (ideally 16°C to 20°C or 60.8°F to 68°F) aligns with the natural drop in body temperature and supports better sleep quality.

Chapter Nine

Building Resilience

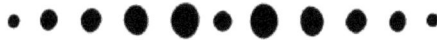

• • • ● • ● • • • •

Strengthening Your Foundation for Growth and Adaptability

R esilience, as defined by psychologists, is the process of adapting well when faced with adversity, trauma, threats, or significant stress. This adaptation can be physical, psychological, or a combination of both. The journey toward resilience inevitably involves facing distress, which is a critical part of the process.

Understanding and Managing Stress

Stress manifests itself as a physiological phenomenon in our bodies, often showing up as inflammation and a cascade of chemical messages that rush through our system. This reaction pushes our heart rate up, causes us to breathe faster and shallower, and prepares us for a perceived threat, essentially priming us for survival. A key research paper by Jonathan Stone argues that stress induces resilience, designed as part of our evolutionary responses to hostile environments [1]. These environments could include a lack of food, cold stress, or physical exertion. This concept is known as hormesis, which refers to the adaptive response of cells and organisms to moderate and intermittent stress. The idea of hormesis dates to the early 16th-century Swiss scientist and physician Paracelsus, who famously stated:

> "All things are poison, and nothing is without poison; the dose alone makes a thing not poison."

Hormesis suggests that stresses such as exercising outdoors can build muscle and provide much-needed vitamin D, though excessive stress can be harmful, leading to skin damage or hypothermia in the case of cold exposure. However, moderate and intermittent exposure to cold can build resilience, offering positive health benefits and enhancing our ability to manage other stresses in life.

The Science Behind Stress-Induced Resilience

In addition to Stone's work, numerous studies in fields such as neuroscience, sports medicine, cancer research, healthy aging, dementia, Parkinson's disease, and Ophthalmology have reported the benefits of stress-induced resilience. These benefits include faster wound healing and a demonstrable slowing of age-related degeneration in the brain, nervous tissue, muscles, and bones. Essentially, exposure to stress, such as that experienced during a cold shower, can contribute to a longer and healthier life.

A study published in Experimental Physiology showed that swimming exercise decreases depression-like behaviour in diabetic mice by reducing inflammation. According to the authors, this improvement in mood and reduction in inflammation might be a useful treatment for depression-related disorders in patients with type 2 diabetes [2].

Embracing Discomfort

While it might seem counterintuitive to willingly expose ourselves to stress—like taking a cold shower or swimming on a winter's day—these activities offer numerous overlooked benefits. They enhance psychological resilience, which can be applied to various areas of everyday life. When done with appropriate caution and a healthy sense of fear, cold water swimming provides a controlled, safe, yet exciting challenge. It's the perfect environment to experience—and get used to—moments of controlled, measured stress, which can help build resilience.

Imagine diving into icy water. The initial shock is enough to make you gasp, but this very discomfort is what forces your body to adapt. Your heart races, your skin tingles, and your breath quickens. This cascade of physiological responses builds both physical and mental toughness. Over time, you become more comfortable with the discomfort, which translates to greater resilience in other areas of life.

Let's break it down further. Regular exposure to cold water has been shown to improve mood, boost immune function, and increase overall well-being. It's not just about surviving the cold; it's about thriving because of it. The act of willingly stepping into a cold environment can also enhance self-discipline and mental fortitude—qualities that are invaluable when facing life's challenges.

So, how can you integrate these principles into your life? Start with small, manageable challenges and gradually increase the difficulty. Begin with short, cold showers, gradually increasing the duration as you get used to the cold. Engage in outdoor activities, even in less-than-ideal weather, to build physical and mental resilience.

Practice mindfulness and meditation to improve your ability to handle stress. Incorporate physical challenges such as hiking, running, or swimming to push your limits. Maintain a healthy diet, get adequate sleep, and engage in regular physical activity to support overall well-being.

By embracing these strategies and understanding the science behind stress and resilience, you can develop a stronger mindset and body, better equipped to handle life's inevitable challenges.

Remember, cold water swimming isn't just about braving the elements; it's about embracing them. The initial shock might be jarring, but the benefits are profound. The act of deliberately stepping into a cold environment prepares you to face life's challenges head-on.

Embrace the cold, push your boundaries, and you'll find yourself stronger, more resilient, and better equipped to handle whatever life throws your way. So, the next time you're feeling down or just a bit out of sorts, consider taking a plunge into cold water. It might just be the reset button your body and mind need to feel rejuvenated and ready to tackle whatever life throws your way.

Conclusion & Personal Account

To begin, this isn't just my theory but it's one that I whole heartedly support and believe to be true. Firstly, we must understand the connection between inflammation, physical illness, and mental health which we've explored throughout this book. This link supports the theory that activities such as cold-water swimming could be a game-changer for treating depression. The symptoms of depression and the behaviours of physically sick individuals share striking similarities, suggesting a common underlying cause—possibly, and what I believe is inflammation. Understanding what causes inflammation and how cold-water swimming might mitigate it can offer insights into warding off both physical ailments and mental malaise.

Inflammation primarily kicks in as a response to infection and injury, acting as a crucial repair mechanism in the body. But here's the catch: this response, governed by the autonomic nervous system, can also be triggered by chronic stress, fatigue or what we used to call melancholy. Unlike infection and injury, chronic stress doesn't really call for an inflammatory response, making it a problematic condition when it leads to persistent inflammation. For a long time, the traditional medical view was that the autonomic nervous system, since it operates on autopilot, wasn't a suitable target for medical interventions. Thankfully, this perspective is changing, thanks to emerging research showing the success of practices like breathing techniques, meditation, and cold-water swimming in influencing the autonomic nervous system.

The nervous system is divided into two main parts: the somatic and the autonomic. The somatic nervous system is under our conscious control and includes the musculoskeletal system, allowing us to move and interact with our environment. On the other hand, the autonomic nervous system runs the show behind the scenes, regulating functions like heart rate and breathing without any conscious effort from us.

The autonomic nervous system is further split into two parts: the sympathetic and parasympathetic systems. These two are like the yin and yang of our body's stress responses. The sympathetic system is responsible for the "fight or flight" response, ramping up our heart rate, blood pressure, blood sugar, and inflammation. In contrast, the parasympathetic system promotes "rest and digest" functions, bringing down inflammation and helping the body reset. The vagus nerve, which starts at the brainstem, plays a big role in this process, reducing inflammation and aiding recovery.

Modern lifestyles often leave our parasympathetic nervous system a bit sluggish, making us more vulnerable to stress and inflammation. For optimal health, we need to keep both the sympathetic and parasympathetic systems in balance. This is where cold water therapy helps. It engages both systems, providing a balanced workout. Initially, cold exposure triggers a sympathetic response, giving us a boost of alertness and energy. However, with repeated exposure, the body's response adjusts, helping us achieve a more balanced physiological and mental state.

After adapting to the cold, the initial sympathetic boost diminishes, allowing the parasympathetic system to become more active. This promotes recovery and reduces inflammation. Regular cold-water swimmers, those who take cold showers and indulge in the occasional ice bath often report feeling rejuvenated and resilient, with lower levels of anxiety and depression. The initial euphoria from the sympathetic activation is balanced by the long-term calming effects of the parasympathetic response, helping prevent lifestyle-related illnesses.

When we immerse our faces in cold water, the parasympathetic nervous system kicks in, recalibrating the body's natural resting state and lowering the concentration of inflammatory chemicals. This physiological shift helps us feel more like our best selves, both physically and mentally. Cold water swimming, therefore, not only gives us an immediate mood boost but also promotes long-term health by reducing chronic inflammation and enhancing the balance between the sympathetic and parasympathetic systems.

Embrace the cold, push your boundaries, and you'll find yourself stronger, more resilient, and better equipped to handle whatever life throws your way.

"If we always choose comfort we never learn the deepest capabilities of our mind or body – Wim Hof"

Chapter Ten

Frequently Asked Questions

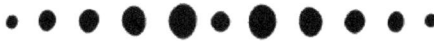

• • • ● ● • ● • • •

1. What are the primary benefits of cold exposure?

> Cold exposure can enhance metabolism, insulin sensitivity, heart health, reduce inflammation, and improve mental resilience.

2. How does cold exposure improve mental health?

> It stimulates the production of norepinephrine, which helps with focus, mood regulation, and stress management.

3. What physiological response helps maintain body temperature in the cold?

Vasoconstriction redirects blood flow from extremities to the core, minimizing heat loss.

4. What is shivering, and why is it significant?

Shivering generates heat through rapid muscle contractions, aiding in maintaining body temperature.

5. What are the risks of hypothermia during cold exposure?

Hypothermia can cause lethargy, weakened heartbeat, and organ failure if not promptly addressed.

6. How can cold-water immersion benefit athletes?

It improves endurance, speeds recovery, and reduces delayed-onset muscle soreness.

7. What is the optimal temperature for a cold plunge?

Between 8-15°C (50-59°F) for therapeutic benefits without causing excessive discomfort.

8. How does cold exposure affect metabolic health?

It boosts HDL cholesterol, improves insulin sensitivity, and aids in glucose metabolism.

9. What is the role of brown adipose tissue (BAT) in cold exposure?

BAT generates heat through non-shivering thermogenesis, aiding in weight management and metabolic health.

10. Can cold exposure help prevent Type 2 diabetes?

Maybe, further research is needed to know conclusively via the process of improving glucose regulation and increasing insulin sensitivity.

11. How do men and women differ in their response to cold?

Men and women differ in their response to cold primarily due to variations in body composition, metabolic rate, hormonal influences, and blood flow, with men generally tolerating cold better while women feel it more intensely in extremities.

12. What are the benefits of winter workouts?

They enhance cardiovascular efficiency, prevent overheating, and support better oxygen uptake.

13. What precautions should be taken during cold-weather exercise?

Dress in layers, avoid prolonged exposure, and warm up properly to reduce injury risk.

14. What is RMB3, and how is it linked to cold exposure?

RMB3 is a cold shock protein activated by cold exposure, potentially protecting against neurodegenerative diseases.

15. How can cold-water swimming improve mental health?

It boosts mood through endorphin release, reduces depression, and enhances resilience.

16. What are the safety tips for cold-water swimming?

Gradual acclimatization, wearing proper gear, and swimming with a group are essential for safety.

17. How does cold exposure aid in menopause symptom management?

Cold-water swimming can reduce hot flashes, anxiety, and mood swings in menopausal women.

18. What are the mental benefits of cold-water swimming?

It alleviates stress, boosts self-esteem, and fosters a sense of community.

19. How does cold exposure help with pain management?

It reduces inflammation and numbs sensory nerves, providing pain relief.

20. What is contrast therapy?

Alternating between hot and cold exposure, it aids in recovery, improves circulation, and reduces inflammation.

21. How does cold exposure influence cardiovascular health?

It improves blood pressure and circulation by training blood vessels to adapt to temperature changes.

22. What is the "after-drop" phenomenon in cold-water swimming?

After-drop occurs when core body temperature continues to fall after exiting cold water.

23. What preparation is needed for cold-water swimming?

Gradual exposure, proper equipment, and initial practice in warmer months are recommended.

24. What role does norepinephrine play in cold exposure?

It enhances focus, mood, and resilience, contributing to stress management.

25. Why is cold-water swimming beneficial for respiratory health?

Regular swimmers report fewer respiratory tract infections due to improved immune response.

References

Embracing the Cold

1. M. Barwood, J. Corbett and C. Wagstaff, "Habituation of the Cold Shock Response May Include a Significant Perceptual Component," Aviation Space Environmental Medicine, vol. 85, no. 2, pp. 167-71, 2014.

2. S. Kwiecien and M. McHugh, "The Cold Truth: The Role of Cryotherapy in the Treatment of Injury and Recovery from Exercise," European Journal Applied Physiology, vol. 121, no. 8, pp. 2125-2142, 2021.

3. M. Eimonte, N. Eimantas, L. Daniuseviciute, H. et al, Brazaitis, "Recovering Body Temperature from Acute Cold Stress is Associated with Delayed Proinflammatory Cytokine Production in Vivo," Cytokine, pp. 143-155, 2021.

Transformative Effects of the Cold

1. van Marken Lichtenbelt, et al, "Healthy Excursions outside the Thermal Comfort Zone," Building Research & Information, pp. 819-827, 2017.

2. Schulz TJ, Tseng YH., "Brown Adipose Tissue: Development, Metabolism and Beyond," Biochem J 15 July 2013; 453 (2): 167–178, pp. 167-178, 2013.

3. Kasiphak Kaikaew, et al, "Sex Difference in Cold Perception and Shivering Onset Upon Gradual Cold Exposure," Journal of Thermal Biology, pp. 137-146, 2018.

4. van den Beukel, J.C., Grefhorst, A. et al, "Women have More Potential to Induce Browning of Perirenal Adipose Tissue than Men". Obesity, 23: 1671-1679. 2015.

Winter Wellness

1. Tyler CJ, Reeve T, Hodges GJ, Cheung SS, "The Effects of Heat Adaptation on Physiology, Perception and Exercise Performance in the Heat: A Meta-Analysis," Sports Medicine, p. 1699–1724, 2016.

2. V. M. Lichtenbelt, H. M. W., H. Pallubinsky, B. Kingma and L. Schellen, "Healthy Excursions outside the Thermal Comfort Zone," Building Research & Information, pp. 819-827, 2017.

3. E. Calton, M. Soares and A. James, "The Potential Role of Irisin in the Thermoregulatory Responses to Mild Cold Exposure in Adults," American Journal of Human Biology, pp. 699-704, 2016.

4. C. J. Stevens, K. A, S. D, et al, "Running Performance in the Heat is Improved by Similar Magnitude with Pre-Exercise Cold-Water Immersion and Mid-Exercise Facial Water Spray," Journal of Sports Science, vol. 35, no. 8, pp. 798-805, 2017.

5. J. Heydenreich, K.. et. al, "Effects of Internal Cooling on Physical Performance, Physiological & Perceptional Parameters when Exercising in the Heat," Frontiers in Physiology, pp. 11-14, 2023.

Cold Water Swimming

1. van Tulleken C, Tipton M, Massey H, Harper CM, "Open Water Swimming as a Treatment for Major Depressive Disorder," British Medical Journal, 2018.

2. The Guardian, "Could Cold Water Swimming Help Treat Depression?," 13 September 2018. [Online, Accessed 14 April 2024].

3. Massey H, Gorczynski P, Harper CM, et al, "Perceptive Impact of Outdoor Swimming on Heath: Web-Based Survey," Interactive Journal of Medical Research, pp. 1-15, 2022.

4. M. Gibas-Dorna, Z. Chęcińska, E. Korek, J. Kupsz, A. Sowińska and H. Krauss, "Cold Water Swimming Beneficially Modulates Insulin Sensitivity in Middle-Aged Individuals," Journal Aging Physical Activity, pp. 547-554, 2016.

5. Knechtle B, Waśkiewicz Z, Sousa CV, Hill L, Nikolaidis PT., "Cold Water Swimming-Benefits and Risks: A Narrative Review," International Journal of Environmental Research Public Health, pp. 1-20, 2020.

6. Manolis AS, Apostolaki N, Melita H et al, "Winter Swimming: Body Hardening and Cardiorespiratory Protection Via Sustainable Acclimation," Current Sports Medicine Reports, pp. 401-415, 2019.

7. Bastide, A., Peretti, D., Knight, J. R., Grosso, S.,& al, e.l. "RTN3 Is a Novel Cold-Induced Protein and Mediates Neuroprotective Effects of RBM3." *Current Biology*, Vol 27, 638-650, 2017.

8. Peretti, D., Bastide, A., Radford, H., & al, el.. "RBM3 Mediates Structural Plasticity and Protective Effects of Cooling in Neurodegeneration." *Nature*, 236-239. 2015.

9. Peretti, D., Smith, H., Verity, N., & al, el. "TrkB Signalling Regulates the Cold-Shock Protein RBM3-Mediated Neuroprotection." *Life Science Alliance*, 1-16. 2021.

10. Van Pelt DW, Hettinger ZR, Dupont-Versteegden EE. "Cold Shock RNA-Binding Protein RBM3 as a Potential Therapeutic." *Journal of Orthopaedics and Orthopaedic Surgery*, 30-34. 2020.

The Benefits of Cold-Water Swimming for Women

1. N. Santoro, "Perimenopause: From Research to Practice," *Journal of Women's Health Vol. 25, No. 4,* vol. 25, no. 4, pp. 332-339, 2016.

2. Troìa, L., Martone, S., Morgante, G., & Luisi, S. "Management of Perimenopause Disorders: Hormonal Treatment," *Gynaecological Endocrinology*, vol. 27, no. 3, pp. 195-200, 2021.

3. Pound M, Massey H, Roseneil S, et al, "How Do Women Feel Cold Water Swimming Affects their Menstrual and Perimenopausal Symptoms?," Post Reproductive Health, vol. 30, no. 1, pp. 11-27, 2024.

4. Gundle. L, Atkinson A, "Pregnancy, Cold Water Swimming and Cortisol: The Effect of Cold Water Swimming on Obstetric Outcomes," *Medical Hypotheses,* vol. 144, no. 1, 2020.

5. Minkin MJ, "Menopause: Hormones, Lifestyle, and Optimizing Aging," *Obstetrics and Gynaecology Clinics of North America,* vol. 46, no. 3, pp. 501-514, 2019.

Cryotherapy & Contrast Therapy

1. T. R. Higgins, D. Greene and M. Baker, "Effects of Cold Water Immersion and Contrast Water Therapy for Recovery From Team Sport: A Systematic Review and Meta-Analysis," Journal of Strength and Conditioning Research, pp. 1443-1460, 2017.

2. Srámek. P, Simecková. M, et al, "Human Physiological Responses to Immersion into Water of Different Temperatures," European Journal of Applied Physiology 81, 436–442 (2000)., pp. 436-442, 2000.

3. Peake. JM, Markworth. JF, Cumming KT, et al, "The Effects of Cold Water Immersion and Active Recovery on Molecular Factors That Regulate Growth and Remodelling of Skeletal Muscle After Resistance Exercise," Frontiers in Physiology, 2020.

4. J. W. Myrer, D. Draper and E. Durrant, "Contrast Therapy & Intramuscular Temperature in the Human Leg," Journal of Athletic Training, pp. 318-322, 1994.

5. A. Buijze, i. Siereveit, B. Heijden and M. F.-D. M. Dijkgraaf, "The Effect of Cold Showering on Health & Work: A Randomized Controlled Trail," Plos One, 2016.

Embracing Seasonal Changes for Better Sleep

1. Feinberg, L. "Topographic Differences in the Adolescent Maturation of the Slow Wave EEG during NREM Sleep, During NREM Sleep. Sleep", *Sleep Research Society*, 325-333, 2011.

2. Schmitt, B. "Sleep and Epilepsy Syndromes", Neuropediatrics, 171–180, 2015.

3. Lucey BP, McCullough A, Landsness EC, Toedebusch CD, McLeland JS, Zaza AM, Fagan. "Reduced Non-Rapid Eye Movement Sleep is Associated with Tau Pathology in Early Alzheimer's Disease". *Science Translational Medicine*, 1-28, 2019.

4. Priano L, Bigoni M, Albani G, Sellitti L, Giacomotti E, et al. "Sleep Microstructure in Parkinson's Disease: Cycling Alternating Pattern (CAP) as a Sensitive Marker of Early NREM". *Sleep Medicine*, 57-62, 2019.

5. Rochette AC, Soulières I, Berthiaume C, Godbout R. "NREM Sleep EEG Activity and Procedural Memory: A Comparison Between Young Neurotypical and Autistic Adults Without Sleep Complaints". *Autism Research: Official Journal of the International Society for Autism Research*, 613–623, 2018.

6. Margri J C, Xuereb, S et al. "Sleep Measures and Cardiovascular Disease in Type 2 Diabetes Mellitus". Clinical Medicine, 380-6, 2023.

7. .Pan, L., Zhiwei, L., & Lan, L. "Investigation of Sleep Quality Under Different Temperatures Based on Subjective and Physiological Measurements". *Science and Technology for the Built Environment*, 1030-1043, 2011.

8. Pan, L., Zhiwei, L., & Lan, L. "Investigation of Sleep Quality Under Different Temperatures Based on Subjective and Physiological Measurements". *Science and Technology for the Built Environment*, 1030-1043, 2011.

9. Tamás, H. "Temperature Exposure and Sleep Duration: Evidence from Time Use Surveys". *Economics and Human Biology*, 1-12, 2024.

Building Resilience

1. Stone J, Mitrofanis J, Johnstone DM, et al. "Acquired Resilience: An Evolved System of Tissue Protection in Mammals." *Dose-Response*. 2018;16(4)

2. Gilak-Dalasm M, Peeri M, Azarbayjani MA. "Swimming Exercise Decreases Depression-like Behaviour and Inflammatory Cytokines in a Mouse Model of type 2 diabetes." Exp Physiol. 1981-1991,2021